# Neural Tube Defects

# Neural Tube Defects

## Jorge A Lazareff
*University of California Los Angeles, USA*

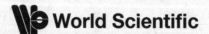

**World Scientific**

NEW JERSEY · LONDON · SINGAPORE · BEIJING · SHANGHAI · HONG KONG · TAIPEI · CHENNAI

*Published by*

World Scientific Publishing Co. Pte. Ltd.

5 Toh Tuck Link, Singapore 596224

*USA office:* 27 Warren Street, Suite 401-402, Hackensack, NJ 07601

*UK office:* 57 Shelton Street, Covent Garden, London WC2H 9HE

**British Library Cataloguing-in-Publication Data**
A catalogue record for this book is available from the British Library.

ISBN-13 978-981-4273-84-8
ISBN-10 981-4273-84-8

Typeset by Stallion Press
Email: enquiries@stallionpress.com

Printed in Singapore.

Publishers' page

*To Barbara van de Wiele, M.D.*

# Contents

# Chapter 1

# Introduction

Neural tube defects (NTD) are the most common disabling congenital malformations. Three hundred thousand individuals are born each year with NTD. It is safe to state that every pediatrician will be involved in the care of children with NTD more often than children with brain tumor.

The neural tube is the primordial structure of the central nervous system. The brain and the spinal cord will develop from the neural tube, guided by a delicate and ill-defined interaction between genes and the environment. This process transforms a flat slab of tissue, the neuroectoderm, into a hollow structure that at one stage stretches along the full length of the embryo. Eventually the neural tube will fade after it is completed.

At term the brain and the spinal cord will be fully formed while none of the original components of the neural tube is identifiable in the newborn. This is true for most people, except for a small but persistent number of individuals (year after year, since the dawn of recorded history), who will carry an anatomical anomaly resulting from an imperfect closure of their neural tubes.

A neural tube is defective when it fails to close between 18 and 28 days following conception. The problem can be anywhere along its structure and according to the location of the opening, the child will have one of a gamut of pathologies that ranges from simple to fatal, from spina bifida to anencephaly, from mild to severe. As the defect happens in a short but crucial moment of development, some patients will have different associated anomalies and others will not, thus highlighting the protean manifestations of NTD. The physician who has been told that a child with any of the NTD conditions will be transferred to his/her care has to be prepared for a few scenarios and leave space for the unexpected. Each patient with NTD is a unique clinical case that will capture the attention of an inquisitive physician.

The etiology or etiologies behind the development of NTD remain ill defined. Prevention through a daily dose of folic acid by the mother before conception has decreased its incidence substantially, but still it has not eradicated the condition. It is a mistake to presume that dietary supplementation of folic acid is enough to prevent this congenital anomaly.

In the developing countries, the incidence of children born with NTD is double or triple than the incidence in the industrialized nations. The difference in incidence also follows the pattern of the poverty line. In Guatemala, the incidence of NTD is 1.6 per 1000 live births; the only places where this figure is similar to the US are few hospitals in the privileged zones of Guatemala City. In contrast, the prevalence of NTD in Quiche, a rural and backward region of the country, is one of the highest in the world. And this difference in Guatemala cannot be attributed alone to prenatal diagnosis that leads to elective abortion.

Interestingly, there is also a different attitude towards the disease. In the US, which has prevalence below the world average, there is an effective healthcare facility available for taking care of children born with NTD. Conversely, more often than not, the parents of a child born with NTD in Guatemala or Kenya are told that their child's condition has a guarded prognosis and is tantamount to immediate demise. These beliefs have led to the accepted practice of sending the child home under the care of their parents, in a great number of nations. Finally when the child has tenaciously continued to live, the family will start a sort of "pilgrimage" between various medical centers that will exhaust their resources and stamina. Thus a child in a developing nation, who has survived the initial brunt of being born with NTD will continue to survive, plagued by preventable complications and thus will be unable to achieve his or her expected intellectual abilities. In Guatemala, 90% of children born with NTD die in the first five months of life. Even if only 10% of the untreated children survive, they represent an increasing number of population who have been virtually neglected by society. It is believed that in rural areas of developing countries, the mortality can reach 100%.

This clearly shows that depending on the location where such a child with NTD is born, its clinical outcome is apt to vary. The scenario in developed nations are different with tremendous resources being allocated to improvement of healthcare.

Furthermore, current US President Barrack Obama has raised the question on how much investment a nation can afford in improvement of healthcare. Following this argument, distinguished thinkers such as Peter Singer have advocated for a dispassionate definition of futility that necessary leads to asking the true worth of human life, the latter defined not by the needs of the individual but by the needs of the society that nestles him/her.

In March 2005, Drs Eduardo Verhagen and Pieter Sauer from the University Medical Center in Groningen, the Netherlands, published in the *New England Journal of Medicine* the protocol for neonatal euthanasia. They report that in a way neonatal euthanasia had been prevalent in their country for decades. By proposing a set of rules to be followed by physicians and parents, the authors acknowledge that the situation they are describing is more real than the society is ready to accept. The Groningen protocol focuses only on perceived or potential suffering by the newborn, it does not ever mention national economic resources as an argument for their position. Nonetheless, in an article in the *Los Angeles Times* in March 2006, Peter Singer linked neonatal euthanasia to the stress of healthcare budget by highlighting that infant mortality in the Netherlands was much less than in the US. Singer attributed this difference to the better management of resources in the US.

In any case, the set of instructions developed by European neo-natologists remind us that the subjective perception that patients with disorders of the brain or the cord are less recoverable than any other patient is more prevalent than we want to admit.

As briefly mentioned above, elective abortion of the child with antenatal diagnosis of NTD could be a cause of the decrease in its prevalence in other nations. Jonathan Glover in *"Causing Death and Saving Lives"* reproduces a letter to the editor of *Times* from a parent of a child born with spina bifida. A part of the text reads, "Why can one kill perfectly well babies by abortion and yet if they are actually born (but turn out wrongly) insist they live, even to the extent of operations, incubators and oxygen tents?"

The reference to this debate is pertinent to this book because the great majority of euthanized neonates in the Netherlands had spina bifida. Any patient with NTD, either because of mental retardation or dependence to a wheelchair or a ventriculoperitoneal shunt for hydrocephalus, represents one of the three groups of elective patients defined in the Groningen protocol: "infants with a hopeless prognosis who experience what parents and experts deem to be unbearable suffering". The authors acknowledge that this group is difficult to define but serve us the example of "a child with the most serious form of spina bifida".

For the moment, until the debate becomes part of public policy, it is patently clear that in the industrialized nations we still take a proactive position with our patients with NTD. We approach them with the same impetus as we do with other patients with cardiac or renal chronic disorders.

But it has to be acknowledged that while we may not be ready yet to let the budget rule the way we treat our patients, we have become accustomed to linking economy to healthcare needs, even if that is done bypassing human rights in the process.

The Western nations have been rightly protesting the lack of medical treatment for patients with AIDS in sub-Saharan Africa. Former South African President Thabo Mbeki has been ridiculed by his stance on the origin and treatment of AIDS. In contrast, the Western advocates for global health have not raised the issue of patients with NTD, perhaps because as mentioned above, we have accepted that in developing nations the needs of patients with NTD are prioritized according to the available budget.

Perhaps, when hearing of a developing nation, some readers may have a limited idea of what it means. The boundary between a country about which we are aware through the daily news because of deep unrest, and a country that while struggling against economical odds has not slid into chaos is not always well traced. To continue with the case of Guatemala, this is a nation with a gross national product of 48 billion US dollars. The nation is not prosperous by industrialized standards but neither has it sunk into an economical void. But still, only 10% of the children with NTD survive up to five months of age.

The current situation demands a solution and it could come by adopting one of the following three options:

1. Improve prevention and treatment of NTD.
2. Implement the Groningen Protocol for euthanasia of the severely ill newborns.
3. Continue the status quo.

The first alternative implies that physicians understand that their patients have similar chance of recovery and improvement as any other subgroup of pathologies. Patients who have cancer or chronic infectious disease will not fare better than patients with NTD if they are abandoned to their fate. A group of devoted physicians can start a spina bifida clinic. Eventually the project will grow. There are international NGO and healthcare agencies that can finance the project. The accumulated experience by a single group of physicians that follows patients whose defects were corrected at different stages of the patients' lives will provide valuable information about the natural history of NTD and its associated conditions.

There are two compelling arguments in favor of transforming NTD into a subject of interest for healthcare officials of a developing nation.

First, the number of working hours that the family spends every year by going back and forth between skeptic physicians of various specialties who cannot solve preventable complications are wasted time for the national economy. I have had the opportunity to participate in numerous clinical and surgical workshops in many countries and I have witnessed, and admired, the determination of the parents of children with NTD who persistently travel to the capital, attracted by the news of a team of foreign doctors laboring with their local colleagues. If the parents of a child with spina bifida from Guatemala feel that everything possible was done for their handicapped child they will carry on with their life and work with the same relief that any other parent from an industrialized nation will feel. The children with the disability will have limited educational opportunities and this will deepen their dependence and indirectly the dependence of their families.

Second, the equipment required for the majority of NTD reparative surgeries is not more sophisticated than the ones required for an abdominal surgery. More often than not, the elements for solving the problem are present but remain idle. Equipping a hospital and training doctors for addressing many NTD conditions in the newborn will improve the medical care of other conditions besides NTD.

The euthanasia of the newborn according to the Groningen Protocol will require a daunting effort from the physicians and the families, and even a debate in the legislative branch of goverment. The idea, to the best of my understanding, is impracticable. There may be a group of parents who wish that their children were dead, and although I have seen many children with NTD who were abandoned by their families, all were left behind in places where they could be easily found and were swaddled in warm clothes.

Leaving things as they are will perpetuate a problem. And in essence this is a moral fallacy. Euthanasia is also performed by nature but not everybody dies. Eighty percent of the children born everyday do so in developing nations, where NTD have a higher incidence than in their industrialized counterparts. So while the government of a developing nation acknowledges the problem by enforcing fortification, it has been shown that the prevalence of NTD does not zero the incidence; while multiple issues regarding prevention are being implemented and perfected, children with NTD continue to be born. The problem is here today for 300,000 families every year.

Virchow declared that medicine is a social science, thus it is reasonable to infer that the physician is a social worker. This mantle does not cover only the general practitioner, or the public health official; it encompasses every physician who is devoted to treating complex diseases, independently of their prevalence.

The neurosurgeons, the geneticist and every one of the specialists who work with patients with NTD are immersed in the struggles of the society where they live, even if some presume that they are not. It goes without saying that patients, their families and their physicians are members of the same society. They all know that a newborn with neural tube defects represents a formidable challenge for the healthcare system of any nation. When basic care is provided the conditions are rarely fatal, therefore the shape and weight of the problems that the physicians will have to confront will vary according to regions of the world.

The truth is that in the great majority of the countries in the world, there are facilities for looking after a wide array of pathologies associated with NTD. I have visited and worked in public hospitals in nations from every continent and everywhere I found teams of physicians absolutely capable of tackling the most complex case of NTD.

It is even fair to state that the difference between developed and underdeveloped nation is less wide when we compare the quality of the physicians at both sides of the divide. I have also witnessed that the enthusiasm of many is slashed every day by the realities of society. And here we return to the question indirectly posed by Virchow, is the physician an agent of social change?

Some authors believe that the doctor has to be devoted to his patient and not be preoccupied with philosophical activism, of which politics is one of its branches. Fair enough, so what can we do to face the challenges posed by our patients?

It has been estimated that the cost of treating a child with spina bifida is close to US$350,000. The elements of this enormous expense are education and medical care. Certainly a child who never had an infection, only one shunt for hydrocephalus, and who had adequate care for urological and orthopedic complications will represent one end of the curve. The benefits of adequate treatment and prevention can be quantified in dollars. Let us reduce the suffering of each of our patients with the understanding that we will be improving the national healthcare budget — a proposition that seems inadequate for a physician, but it is the language that administrators and politicians understand and the benefit for all the patients will be immense. This can be achieved without surrendering any of our principles as physicians.

It is the purpose of this handbook to provide an encompassing review of the clinical aspects of all neural tube defects. The text is succinct but not basic and is centered on the clinical neurosciences because NTD is, above all, pathology of the central nervous system. The details of the different surgical techniques are mentioned to facilitate the understanding of the pathology.

When writing this book we had in mind the pediatrician and general practitioners who practice anywhere in the world and mostly from rural areas where patients with neural tube defects are born at a rapid pace every day.

**Chapter 2**

# Pathogenesis

The complexity of the vertebrate nervous system stems from its even complex embryogenesis which by and large has seemed to be preserved among different vertebrates. The epicenter of the kaleidoscope lies on a distinct group of cells in the dorsal ectoderm which has a diametrically different fate. This group of cells gets segregated from the rest of the ectodermal cells by a process called *neural induction* and this prepares the ground for receiving a myriad of signals from within the genetic makeup of the embryo itself, and it thus transforms itself into the neural tube through a highly regulated process. This transformation process is called *neurulation* and the segregated group of cells called *neural plate*, with *neural induction* the mechanism by which the neural plate is formed.

Although the quest for this neural inducing signal stretched slightly over seven decades, yet the modern knowledge of this intricate process comes from the contribution of two German Scientists, namely Spemann and Mangold, whose pioneering work came from experiments involving amphibian embryos. Some important facts from this groundbreaking study are described here.

The two most significant contributions in understanding the development of the vertebrate nervous system are the discoveries of the organizer and mechanism of its action in neural induction, along with its molecular mechanism that comes from the studies involving amphibian embryos (salamander and Xenopus embryos).

Induction is classically defined as the process by which action of one set of tissue alters or changes the action or fate of another tissue which will have a striking consequences on the tissue induced. The process of neural induction takes place during the gastrulation phase of embryogenesis. According to Spemann and Mangold, the organizer of this neural induction process has the ability to induce the dorsal mesoderm and pattern the remaining mesoderm along with formation of the neuroectoderm.

## Explaining neural induction at the molecular level

Although remarkable information has been gathered regarding the origin of the neural inducing tissues and the timing of these inducing signals, what is yet to be determined is the exact identity of these inducing signals. The concept of a default pathway in which the cells are destined to form neural ectoderm with inhibition of non-neural pathway within the ectoderm is the most plausible explanation. The discovery of Spemann's organizer represents a noteworthy step in the understanding of this complex issue of neural induction. Formation of the neural plate involves induction of dorsal midline ectoderm, or also called the *neuroepithelium*, into the neural plate. At this stage it is the bone morphogenic proteins (BMP) that prevent the default fate of the ectoderm to form neuroectoderm; instead with the help of BMP, epithelium is formed. Thus it has been hypothesized that the BMP signaling pathway specifies ectodermal cells as epithelium but on the other hand its inhibition leads to neural induction. Both BMP-2 and BMP-4 belong to the triple gene block (TGB) super family and is expressed in the ventral part of the embryo where their prime antagonists such as noggin, chordin, and the follistatin which are emanating from the primitive node prevent the default fate of the ectoderm to form neuroectoderm and instead forms the epidermis or cutaneous ectoderm. Another unique ability of the BMP signaling pathway is its ability to interact with other signaling pathways like the fibroblast growth factor family and the WNT family of molecules. With this, we proceed towards an in-depth description of the neurulation process.

## Neurulation

Neurulation is the primary embryonic process that leads to the formation of the neural tube which represents the future brain and the spinal cord. It takes place in two distinct phases, namely primary and secondary neurulation, with each phase representing a complex interplay of genetic and environmental interactions. The process of neurulation, or rather, the process of neural induction, commences with the formation of the neural plate.

## Primary neurulation

This is the main process by which the brain and the spinal cord, up to the level of lower lumbar segments are formed and it occurs between week 3 and 4 of embryonic period. This process is further divided into four steps:

i.   Formation of neural plate
ii.  Shaping of neural plate
iii. Bending of neural plate
iv.  Closure of neural groove

### i. Formation of neural plate

By the process of neural induction, a thickened region of neural plate is formed located medially within the embryo. The process of thickening is by virtue of apicobasal elongation of ectodermal cells with resultant pseudo-stratification and is not due to increase in cell number.

### ii. Shaping of neural plate

During this process the neural plate undergoes alteration in its shape, from being short and flat to assuming a longer and narrower configuration. This is the result of a combination of the following events which takes place in succession:

- Continued apicobasal cell elongation.
- Convergent extension movements resulting in narrower neural plate.
- Cell division with placement of daughter cells along the length of the plate.
- Normal gastrulation movements with caudal ward regression of primitive streak.

### iii. Bending of neural plate

This is a complicated process involving two distinct aspects of movements, namely furrowing and folding.

*Furrowing*: This involves the process of creating three hinge points: the single median hinge point with two paired dorsolateral hinge points, where the actual movement of folding takes place. Furrowing takes place by the phenomenon of wedging, which is apical constriction with basal expansion. The result is the formation of a furrow. There are medial and lateral hinges at the spinal level while there are no lateral hinges in the forebrain. This is mentioned to highlight that cranial malformation of the neural tube might not result from identical process as their spinal counterpart.

*Folding*: This is a slightly more complicated process involving forces generated from adjacent non-neural ectoderm as the cells undergo the process of apicobasal flattening (the opposite of wedging). This allows for rapid expansion of neural folds; [Schoenwolf and Alvarez].

### iv.  Closure of neural groove

This is the last but not the least part of the concert which started with plain thickening of the neural plate. Now the neural plate has turned into a furrow whose ultimate shape will be that of a hollow tube. This process involves the bending of the groove to approximate the neural fold across the midline and thus later attach and fuse. The process is not only very intricate but also highly precise, which requires the interplay of many molecules mediating cell adhesion, epithelial breakdown and lastly fusion. Many of the control mechanisms for this phenomenon are yet to be fully understood.

For many years it was maintained that the closure of the neural tube had a single starting point and proceeded in zip-like fashion caudally and rostrally. The current opinion amongst embryologists is that the neural tube closes from the confluence of three to five initiation areas. The prevalent theory is that forwarded in 1993 by van Allen *et al*. According to them, the site 1 (arbitrary numeration) between apposing neural folds takes place at the rhomboencephalon-spinal cord junction, site 2 starts at the prosencephalon-mesencephalon junction, site 3 begins at the rostral tip of the neural plate, site 4 is between sites 1 and 2 while site 5 is at the caudal end of the neural grove and from there proceeds cranially to meet site 1. Sites 1, 2 and 4 proceed bidirectionally; sites 3 and 5 move unidirectionally, caudally 3 and cephalically 5.

The merit of van Allen was to move embryologist and clinicians away from the concept of a "zip up and down" phenomenon and highlight the complexity of the closure of the neural tube. The current prevailing theory maintains the presence of three closure sites which are basically similar to sites 1, 2 and 3 of the five-site closure theory. Specifically, site 1 is at the hindbrain/cervical boundary, site 2 at the forebrain/midbrain boundary and site 3 at the extreme rostral end of the forebrain.

It has been noted that different mouse strains have different locations for site 2. In some strains it is found caudally to the midbrain while in others it is found rostrally in the forebrain. This variable occurrence of closure 2 could have some pathological significance; in effect, the "caudal" site 2 is less prone to *exencephaly*. When site 1 fails to close, the entire neural tube remains open. This condition is called *craniorachischisis* and is not compatible with life. Failure of closure 3 leads to *anencephaly*. Certainly this commonly seen NTD could be considered as partial defects in closure.

## Secondary neurulation

This process forms the lower cord segments, namely the sacral and the coccygeal segments, by the retrogressive differentiation of the caudal cell mass.

The neural tube is formed in the caudal eminence without neural folding. Mesenchymal cells in the dorsal part of the tail bud form the secondary neural tube that has a continuous lumen with the neural tube formed by primary neurulation.

The anomalies of this process may give rise to closed forms of spina bifida, also called *dysraphic conditions*. Here the developing spinal cord fails to separate from other tissues derived from other embryonary layers.

The common pathological events known to interfere with embryological formation of neural tube are:

1. Maternal folic acid deficiency
2. Maternal diabetes
3. Maternal antiepileptic medications
4. Maternal risk factors

## 1.   Maternal folic acid deficiency

Although NTD are multifactorial in origin, but among the environmental factors, lack of folate has been consistently shown to be related to NTD. Even then the exact mechanism by which folic acid prevents NTD is not very clear.

### Folic Acid Background

Folate is a water soluble vitamin which is abundant in leafy vegetables. The word "folate" derives from the Latin word *"folium"* for leaf. A single proton differentiates folate from its synthetic form, folic acid. The latter is more stable and thus more appropriate for manufacturing into tablets. It is recommended that women consume 0.4 mg supplement in addition to eating food rich in folate. It is presumed that folate is important for DNA metabolism and repair, probably through the following:

## Mechanism of Action

Folic acid needs to be converted into tetrahydrofolate (THF) and then into 5-methyltetrahydrofolate (5-MeTHF) glutamate which is taken into the bloodstream. Inside the cell, folate is an acceptor and donor of one carbon unit and is involved in methylation of DNA, proteins and lipids. In essence, it is accurate to state that folate is essential for cellular function.

When there is a deficit in 5-MeTHF and vitamin $B_{12}$, homocysteine accumulates in the cell. This will result in an increase in S-adenosylhomo-cysteine which will lead to a dysregulation of gene expression for lipid and protein metabolism. An interesting line of research has been derived from this. It has been reported that there are cases where mothers who had adequate folate intake still delivered NTD children, thus emphasizing the role of genetics as a contributing factor in the developing of NTD.

Nonetheless, the epidemiological data about the relation between folate ingest and NTD development is very strong, if not overwhelming. Based on two randomized control trials and several other studies, the US Centers for Disease Control (CDC) made a recommendation in 1992 that all women capable of becoming pregnant should consume 0.4 mg of folic acid per day to reduce the risks of NTDs. In addition, those women who have had a child with a neural tube defect are recommended to consume 4.0 mg when they are attempting pregnancy and during the first trimester.

The two randomized control trials mentioned in the recommendation included the British Medical Research Council (MRC) Vitamin Study and preliminary results from a Hungarian randomized controlled trial of multivitamin/mineral supplementation. The MRC study found that administration of 4.0 mg of folic acid decreased the risk of NTD by 70% in women with a previous NTD affected pregnancy. Women in this study were randomized to receive placebo, folic acid alone, other vitamins without folic acid, or folic acid in addition to other vitamins. The rates of NTDs were significantly higher in the groups that did not receive folic acid. In addition, folic acid plus other vitamins did not decrease the risk of NTDs more than folic acid alone.

The evidence from the Hungarian randomized control trial was published in December 1992 and confirmed the preliminary results discussed in the CDC recommendation. The results indicated that supplementation with 0.8 mg of folic acid significantly decreased the prevalence of NTDs (22.9 per 1000 in vitamin group vs. 13.3 per 1000 in placebo, $p = 0.02$). This study confirmed that folic acid could decrease the risk of NTDs in women without a history of NTD affected pregnancy.

The data from these randomized control trials in addition to data from previous observational studies illustrated that adequate periconceptional intake of folic acid each day reduces the risk of NTD by 50–72%. The CDC recommendation of 0.4 mg was based on examination of the benefit from various doses of folic acid, collected from both the observational and randomized control trials. Subsequently, data collected as part of the China–US Collaborative Project for Neural Tube Defect Prevention found that administration of 0.4 mg of folic acid daily during the periconceptional period decreased the risk of NTDs by 79% (CI:57, 90) in a province in northern China known to have NTD rates of 5 to 6 per 1000 births. Women who were more than 80% compliant had the greatest risk reduction (CI:62, 94). The study also examined risk reduction associated with 0.4 mg folic acid supplementation in a province in southern China known to have lower rates of NTD (1 per 1000 births). In the southern region, folic acid supplementation resulted in a risk reduction of 41% (CI:3, 64). In this group, more than 80% compliance did not further increase the risk reduction (CI:3, 64).

## Folic Acid Fortification

Following the US Public Health Service recommendation in 1992, the Food and Drug Administration (FDA) mandated that certain grain products be fortified with 0.43 to 1.4 mg of folic acid per pound of product. Mandated fortification was required for enriched flour, bread, rolls and buns, farina, corn grits, cornmeal, rice, and noodle products but does not include whole grain products. The mandate was put into effect in January 1998. In addition to fortification, the FDA recommended two other approaches to improving folic acid consumption: (1) improved dietary habits and (2) use of dietary supplements with folic acid.

Following fortification in the United States, several studies illustrated a significant decline in the incidence of neural tube defects. One study reported a 31% decline in the incidence of spina bifida and a 16% decrease in the incidence of anencephaly. Another study reported a 19% decline in the total of NTD births and a 23% decline in spina bifida births.

Several international studies have reproduced similar results following mandatory fortification. Chile began fortifying wheat flour with folic acid in January 2000. The Latino American Collaborative Study of Congenital Malformations (ECLAMC) monitors neural tube defects in Argentina, Bolivia, Brazil, Chile, Ecuador, Paraguay, Uruguay, and Venezuela. Although other South American countries have also begun fortifying, post-fortification data from ECLAMC are only reported for Chile as they began fortification in 2000 with an estimated intake of 360–400 mcg daily per person. Preliminary data released in 2003 illustrated a statistically significant decrease of 31% in the incidence of NTD births. A more complete analysis conducted in 2005 compared pre-existing trends of NTD rates with post-fortification NTD rates and found a 51% decrease in the prevalence of spina bifida births and a 47% decrease in the prevalence of anencephaly births.

Fortification in Canada became mandatory in 1998. Data collected on NTD prevalence rates between 1993 and 2002 illustrated a 53% decrease in spina bifida and a 38% decrease in anencephaly during full fortification periods. In addition, prior to fortification the eastern provinces had significantly higher rates of NTDs than western provinces. The magnitude of decrease was higher in the eastern provinces with a higher baseline rate of NTDs than in the western provinces with a lower baseline rate. After fortification, there were no significant differences in the rates of NTD between western and eastern provinces.

As fortification efforts spread throughout the world, the level of fortification and which products should be fortified become the focus. In the United States, one suggested effort to increase folic acid consumption among certain high risk groups (namely Latina women) is to fortify corn masa flour. One study modeled the possible benefit of fortifying corn masa flour at a level of 140 mcg folic acid/100 g corn masa flour, with data taken from the National Health and Nutrition Examination Survey (NHANES) 2001–2004. It was estimated that fortification of corn masa flour would have increased daily folic acid intake by 19.9% among Mexican-American women aged 15–44 and 4.2% among non-Hispanic white women in the study sample. This effort would target women at increased risk for NTDs while maintaining a relatively stable intake among the general population.

## Folic Acid Consumption Behaviors

Consuming the recommended amount of folic acid each day is a relatively easy way to prevent NTD. However, a 2002 survey conducted in the United States by the March of Dimes Foundation revealed that only 20% of women knew that folic acid could prevent certain birth defects. In addition, of the women surveyed, only 7% knew that they had to take folic acid *before* becoming pregnant. More recently, the results from the 2005 March of Dimes Gallup survey suggest that only 33% of women polled took a dietary supplement daily. In a separate study, although women aware of the relationship between birth defects and folic acid were twice as likely to report being on a daily folic acid supplement, the total percentage of this group of women taking folic acid daily was similar to the amount of women taking folic acid daily in the March of Dimes (2005) survey.

Studies in the United States and other countries have revealed a wide range in the levels of folic acid awareness and in turn, consumption behavior. The lack of effective education strategies regarding folic acid in many countries is a problem that must be addressed in order to prevent neural tube defects. As a result, many countries have taken steps to increase folic acid consumption among women of childbearing age through health education campaigns.

One study conducted in Mexico assessed folic acid awareness at intervals during a campaign to promote folic acid consumption. During the campaign, they offered 5 mg folic acid supplements to low-income women to be taken once a week — the 5 mg pill was the only prescription of folic acid supplement available at that time in Mexico. At nine months, 44% of the 2200 women interviewed were aware of the benefits of folic acid and 32% were taking folic acid. At 28 months, 51% of the women interviewed were aware of the benefits of folic acid and 44% were taking folic acid.

Two years after the initiation of the campaign there was a significant reduction in the rate of NTD births (1.04/1000 in 1999 to 0.58/1000 in 2001, $p < 0.001$).

In South America, a large survey concluded that only 14.8% of women interviewed had taken a vitamin containing folic acid and only about 1% had taken it appropriately to prevent the occurrence of NTDs. In this study, 2810 postpartum women from 30 hospitals throughout South America were interviewed to explore their awareness of the benefit of periconceptional folic acid. About 42% of the women interviewed reported taking vitamins during pregnancy. When asked to state the name of the vitamin it became apparent that only 22% had actually taken vitamins; the rest naming minerals or other products. Folic acid was only present in 14.8% of the vitamins consumed by the women who reported taking vitamins during their pregnancy. Only 7% of the women who reported taking vitamins and 1.6% of all interviewed women took the vitamins within the first month of pregnancy. However, only 2/3 of the vitamins reported contained folic acid. Therefore, only 1% of those reported taking vitamins in the first month of pregnancy actually took folic acid.

Although fortification and supplementation are being studied widely throughout Central America, little has been done to assess awareness of folic acid and neural tube defects in Guatemala. This is especially important as Guatemala has one of the highest rates of neural tube defects worldwide — with an unequal distribution between the rural and urban populations.

Other countries have also explored knowledge of folic acid, neural tube defects, and folic acid consumption practices in hopes of learning how to target messages to women that would promote more folic acid consumption. A study consisting of two surveys done in the Netherlands found that a campaign aimed at increasing folic acid consumption increased folic acid use during the periconceptional period from 0.8% to 4.4%. Studies in the United Kingdom and Ireland illustrated relatively high levels of folic acid knowledge. However, they found that while many women knew of the benefits of folic acid, no more than 50% took folic acid preconceptionally. These findings parallel the findings in the United States, where women are aware that folic acid is beneficial, but are not aware of the exact timing and have not been recommended to take folic acid periconceptionally.

Studies in Israel, the Mediterranean, and Turkey illustrate dismal levels of folic acid use and awareness. In a study in Israel, 5.5% of the women interviewed had heard of folic acid, only 2.8% had taken folic acid, and only 4 out of the 27 women who took folic acid knew why. In the Mediterranean study, 8.1% started taking folic acid before conception but only 6.9% took folic acid during the entire recommended periconceptional period. Despite the high incidence of NTD in Turkey (31.9 per 10,000), only 22% of women in the study had heard or read of folic acid and only 13% stated that folic acid could prevent birth defects.

Additionally, studies in the United States have also pointed out a lack of folic acid consumption and knowledge among women who had had a previous NTD affected pregnancy. Canfield *et al.* (2002) interviewed 195 mothers of infants with NTD and 233 control mothers. In the case-control study, only 32.7% of the interviewed cases were taking folic acid. At the time of the interview, 32.7% of non-pregnant case women and 25.2% of non-pregnant control women reported regularly consuming multivitamins or folic acid. In addition, folic acid consumption varied significantly across ethnic groups. Spanish speaking Hispanic women (13.5%) reported lower folic acid or multivitamin consumption than English speaking Hispanic women (20.0%) and white women (64.7%). Several other studies have reported lower folic acid consumption behaviors among Latina women than among Caucasian women. This is alarming as women with a prior NTD affected pregnancy and Latina women are at greater risk of having an NTD affected pregnancy. It is important that measures be taken to improve periconceptional folic acid consumption in high risk populations of women in addition to all women of childbearing age.

*The Fumonisin Factor*

In Guatemala the government has pursued a plan of folic acid fortification. As a result there has been a decrease of NTD in the central part of the country but not in the mountains. Initially the disparity was attributed to cultural issues to non-compliance of the regulations. Eventually, it was evidenced that the maize consumed by the indigenous population of the Quiché and surrounding areas was infected with Fumonisin B1 (FB1), a maixe mycotoxin. Fumonisins are produced by the fungus *Fusarium verticilloides*. Fumonisin impairs folic acid metabolism. The hydrolyzed form of FB1 does not. The process by which the maize is treated to transform FB1 into FB1H is called *nixtamalization*. As described by Riley *et al.* in Agricultural Research (2001): "Corn is harvested, dried, and graded as being clean, spoiled, or rotten based on the amount of fungal and insect damage. Then it is bagged for storage. Kernels are removed from the cob and mixed in a ratio of one-third clean, one-third spoiled, and one-third rotten. This mix is added to near-boiling water treated with lime. When the corn is soft enough, the liquid is poured off and the remaining material is a hominy-like slurry that is called *nixtamal*. The nixtamal is then rinsed with water — if it is available." How thoroughly they rinse is critical because water washes out some of the toxins. As noted by the authors, the water supply is crucial. Following the same procedure does not guarantee that the flour will be free of FB1.

## Role of Fumonisins

Fumonisins are a family of toxic and carcinogenic mycotoxins produced by *Fusarium verticilloides*, a common fungal contaminant of maize. The toxin does not cause direct harm to humans albeit it does produce cancer in laboratory rats and sickens horses and pigs.

Fumonisins inhibit ceramide synthase, causing accumulation of bioactive intermediates of sphingolipid metabolism, which interferes with function of membrane proteins including human folate receptor (HFR). Fumonisins have been documented to cause NTD and craniofacial defect in mouse embryos.

High incidence of NTD occurs in regions of the world like Guatemala, South America, and China where substantial consumption of fumonisins has been documented. A recent study in Texas found a significant association between NTD/craniofacial defects and consumption of tortillas during the first trimester.

Henk Blom and collaborators have sketched what is known about folate in their published paper in *Nature Review* (2006). These authors give equal preponderance to genetics and environment as modifiers of folate metabolism. Through either way the decreased alteration of proteins, lipids and other metabolits will lead to altered protein function and altered gene expression, and finally to an imperfect closure of the neural tube.

### Vitamin $B_{12}$

It has been documented that there is an association between low maternal vitamin $B_{12}$ level and increased risk of NTD. Vitamin $B_{12}$ is a component of methionine synthase (MS). Decrease in level of MS influences folate metabolism. Decreased level of folate and decreased level of vitamin $B_{12}$ may increase levels of homocysteine and thus increased level of S-adenosyl homocysteine (SAH). SAH plays an important role in gene expression, cell differentiation, and apoptosis during organogenesis.

Methylation index: SAM/SAH, i.e. S-adenosyl methionine/S-adenosyl homocysteine. As the index of SAM/SAH decreases as seen in deficiency of vitamin $B_1$ folate and vitamin $B_{12}$, methylation of DNA also decreases. The end result is NTD.

Raised homocysteine has two effects — homocysteine acts as a direct embryotoxic agent and indirectly it causes disruption of methylation and increases oxidative stress.

In 2003, Ray and Bloom demonstrated the relationship between increased risk of NTD and low maternal vitamin $B_{12}$ level.

### Role of Vitamin $B_6$

Possibility of an association between vitamin $B_6$ and NTD has been noted.

### Role of Selenium

Selenium is one of the most relevant antioxidant in our diet and glutathionine is one of the most important endogenous antioxidant. Selenium depletion facilitates oxidative conditions by inhibiting methionine adenosyltransferase (MAT). Reduced MAT in turn compromises MAT dependant reaction such as DNA synthesis and hypomethylation, which leads to increased risk of having a baby with NTD.

## 2.  Maternal diabetes

Maternal diabetes has been implicated as the second most common causative factor for occurrence of NTD probably after folic acid deficiency. Experimental models show a strong association of diabetes as a causative factor in caudal regression syndrome. Hyperinsulinemia has been found to be a significant risk factor for Hispanic women in Texas.

## 3.  Maternal antiepileptic medications

There is an increased risk of congenital anomalies including NTD in children born to mothers on chronic antiepileptic drugs (AED). The most common association has been seen with sodium valproate and carbamazapine. The exact mechanism is not known, but the following are possible explanations given for the effect of AED on growing fetuses. It is believed that free radicals are relevant to this process because of the following:

i.   Free radical mediated injury from metabolism of AEDs.
ii.  Genetically deficient enzyme pathways involved in scavenging free radicals.
iii. Overload of free radical scavenging enzymes during AED therapy.

*Prevention of NTD in Pregnant Women with AED*

1. Monotherapy is better than polytherapy.
2. Supplemental extra-strength folic acid — 0.4 to 4 mg/day.
3. Addition of antioxidants like selenium — 200 to 400 $\mu$g/day.

When considering the etiological factors it is always worth remembering the sobering example of not so many years ago when a clear association was found between potato blight in Ireland and the dramatic increase in cases of NTD; it was observed that there has been a decrease in NTD cases even before the implementation of folic acid fortification and concomitantly no decrease of NTD birth was noticed in central California.

Our duties as physicians demand that we encourage women of birth age to consider all the risk factors mentioned above, but we also have to be very careful in not transmitting the impression that it is the parents' fault for the birth of a child with NTD.

## 4. Maternal risk factors

### Maternal Age

NTD are common at the extremes of age.

### Parity

The association between maternal parity and incidence of NTD is stronger than that with maternal age. There is modest increase in risk of NTD in mothers with parity of 3 or more. No clear biological explanation has been found for this association.

### Maternal Metabolic Syndrome

The following conditions are grouped under this syndrome: abdominal obesity, diabetes mellitus or insulin resistence, non-white ethnicity, dyslipidemia, arterial hypertension and elevated serum C-reactive protein. The presence of one or two of the abovementioned conditions increased the risk of NTD. Obesity and diabetes are the most commonly observed factors, individually or associated to each other.

### Maternal Obesity

A BMI of >29 doubles the risk for occurrence of NTD. This has been observed consistently.

### Maternal Febrile Illness

Maternal flu or cold in the first trimester has been associated with two- to three-fold increase in risk for NTD. Also noted was the increased risk of NTD associated with maternal usage of hot tub, sauna or any febrile illness. Hyperthermia is a known neuroteratogen. In experimental animal it affects cell proliferation, migration and programmed cell death.

### Parental Socioeconomic Status (SES)

Higher rate of NTD has been noted in areas with lower socioeconomic status. Some studies were more specific and determined that low maternal education was associated with an elevated risk of NTD in offspring. Now, it goes without saying that this is true, except it is easier to define the extremes of SES than the broad middle class with its multiple subcategories. Most likely the low education level has relevance because the parents may not be aware of folate prophylaxis and poverty exposes the individual to a series of teratogens and malnutrition — the all-encompassing medical condition that is called poverty is the real culprit of NTD and low SES.

### Heavy Metals

Increased concentration of cadmium, lead and mercury in the drinking water did not affect the incidence of NTD in a population living two miles away from polluting factories.

### Recreational Drug

Street drugs and alcohol consumption by the mother does not increase NTD incidence, but cigarette smoke, even second hand, is considered as a potential teratogen.

### Parental Occupation

Certain population-based studies have demonstrated an increased risk of NTD with the following category of occupation in parents:

 i. Welding
 ii. Transport
iii. Healthcare profession — nursing/dentistry
 iv. Agriculture

## Suggested Readings

Blom HJ, Shaw GM, den Heijer M, Finnell RH. Neural tube defects and folate: Case far from closed. *Nat Rev Neurosci* 2006; **7**(9):724–731.

Botto LD, Moore CA, Khoury MJ, Erickson JD. Neural-tube defects. *N Engl J Med* 1999; **341**(20):1509–1519.

Chen CP. Syndromes, disorders and maternal risk factors associated with neural tube defects (III). *Taiwan J Obstet Gynecol* 2008; **47**(2):131–140.

Frey L, Hauser WA. Epidemiology of neural tube defects. *Epilepsia* 2003; **44** Suppl 3:4–13.

Marasas WFO, Riley RT, Hendricks KA *et al.* Fumonisins disrupt sphingolipid metabolism, folate transport, and neural tube development in embryo culture and *in vivo*: A potential risk factor for human neural tube defects among populations consuming fumonisin-contaminated maize. *J Nutr* 2004; **134**:711–716.

Nakatsu T, Uwabe C, Shiota K. Neural tube closure in humans initiates at multiple sites: Evidence from human embryos and implications for the pathogenesis of neural tube defects. *Anat Embryol* 2000; **201**(6):455–466.

24                                    *Neural Tube Defects*

Padmanabhan R. Etiology, pathogenesis and prevention of neural tube defects. *Congenit Anom* 2006; **46**(2):55–67.

Schoenwolf GC, Alvarez IS. Roles of neuroepithelial cell rearrangement and division in shaping of the avian neural plate. *Development* 1989; **106**:427–439.

Chapter 3

# Classification

## Anatomical Classification of Neural Tube Defects

### Cranial defects

- Encephalocele
- Anencephaly
- Iniencephaly

### Spinal defects

#### I.  Open Neural Tube Defect

1.  Myelomeningocele
2.  Hemimyelomeningocele

#### II.  Closed Neural Tube Defect

1.  Meningocele
2.  Lipomyelomeningocele
3.  Diastematomyelia
4.  Neurenteric cyst
5.  Dermal sinus
6.  Caudal regression syndrome
7.  Segmental spinal dysgenesis syndrome
8.  Dorsal enteric fistula
9.  Thick filum terminal syndrome
10.  Terminal myelocystocele

## Embryological Classification

### Cranial defects

1.  Anencephaly
2.  Encephalocele
3.  Iniencephaly

**Spinal defects**

I. **Anomalies of Gastrulation**

- **Disorder of notochord formation**
  1. Caudal regression syndrome
  2. Segmental spinal dysgenesis
- **Disorder of notochord integration**
  1. Dorsal enteric fistula
  2. Neurenteric cyst
  3. Diastematomyelia (split cord malformation)
  4. Dermal sinus

II. **Anomalies of Primary Neurulation**

  1. Myelomeningocele
  2. Lipomyelomeningocele
  3. Meningocele

III. **Combined Anomalies of Gastrulation and Primary Neurulation**

  1. Hemimyelomeningocele

IV. **Anomalies of Secondary Neurulation and Retrogressive Differentiation**

  1. Thick filum terminal
  2. Terminal myelocystocele

# Part I

# Spinal Defects

# Chapter 4

# Myelomeningocele

## Introduction

Myelomeningocele (MMCL) is the most common form of NTD and is also known as spina bifida cystica. With adequate and multidisciplinary approach in managing such cases, the survival of children afflicted with MMCL has changed considerably. However, the success rate of this pathology varies perhaps according to where the child is born. In this chapter we will put emphasis on the description of clinical symptoms that may herald the development of a treatable condition, provided it is diagnosed on time.

MMCL is considered as a defect in primary neurulation resulting from failure of closure of the posterior neuropore. The great majority of the length of the spinal cord develops within physiological limits, except for a segment of the cord which is most commonly the lumbosacral segment, where the observer notes the presence of the exposed neural placode.

The incidence of the defect follows the distribution:

- Lumbar-sacral in 85% of cases
- Thoracic in 10% of cases
- Cervical in 5% of cases

This exposed neural placode with the rudimentary central canal running along its long axis represents the ultimate failure of folding and finally fusion of the neural tube. The lateral wall of the defect is lined by the dura mater which fuses with the fascia and the dysplastic epidermis and dermis. The failure in fusion of the bony lamina and the para-spinal muscles follows suit. At times the sac is elevated from accumulation of cerebrospinal fluid (CSF) between the meningeal layers and the neural placode. The lateral most border of the neural placode has transitional epithelium and is at times highly vascular when it is called *medullovasculosa*, similar to cerebrovasculosa of anencephaly.

The placode (P), the central canal (C) and the medullovasculosa (Mv) are depicted in the picture below.

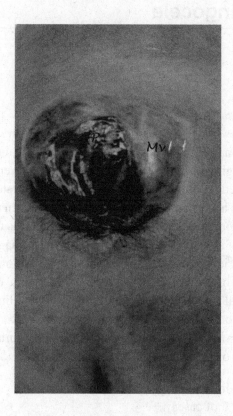

The central groove within the neural placode represents the central canal, wtih the ventral roots exiting medially and the dorsal roots exiting laterally, as it would from the posterior surface of the placode. The junction between the placode and the normal skin is gradual with the dura fusing with the fascia. There is collection of CSF in the subarachnoid space, i.e. between the dura and the neural placode. Functional neural tissue may be present below the placode.

Even if the child presents with a flat defect or bulging protruding sac, in essence both lesions are exactly the same. The bulging sac represents that the CSF has been confined to the defect by a sturdy membrane thus minimizing the deleterious effect of infections from rupture of the sac.

## Incidence

Approximately 3000 pregnancies are affected by MMCL per year in the US. Female preponderance is seen among MMCL-afflicted children. The worldwide incidence of MMCL ranges from 0.17 to 6.39 per 1000 live births.

## Epidemiology

The incidence of MMCL has decreased in industrialized nations. In the US, the 3000 pregnancies mentioned above represent 0.6 per 1000 live births. In rural China and Guatemala, this incidence triples.

## Decline in prevalence

Worldwide, prevalence of MMCL has decreased and one of the reasons could be due to legalization of termination of pregnancies.

Roberts in 1990/1991 reported 23% decline in prevalence of NTD due to medical termination of pregnancy.

Cuckle and Wald reported 31% decline in prevalence of NTD in England and Wales due to termination of pregnancy.

## Impact of folic acid on MMCL

Bol *et al.* proposed from their research that folic acid not only reduces the risk of open NTD but also reduces its severity. Wong and Paulozzi suggested one possible mechanism for reduction of the severity of spina bifida may be that folic acid may move the location of the lesion caudally along the developing spine.

In the pre-fortification era, the incidence of NTD affected pregnancy was approximately 4000 annually. In 1996, folic acid fortification was introduced in the US. Finally in 1998, the folic acid fortification compliance was made mandatory.

The following graph represents the decrease in incidence of NTD in the US. The most recent data shows that the incidence of NTD affected pregnancies is 3000, a decrease by 1000. This phenomenon has been observed in other parts of the world as well.

32                                   *Neural Tube Defects*

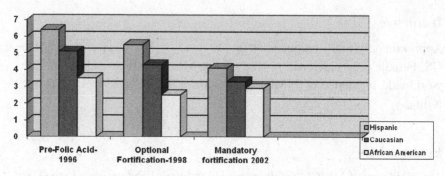

Fig. 1.    Incidence of neural tube defects in the US.

## Racial difference in spite of immigration factors persists

In the US, the incidence of NTD among the different races follows: Hispanics > Caucasians > African Americans > Asians. The incidence for Hispanics is 0.6 per 1000 live birth, while it is 0.23 per 1000 live birth for Asians in the US.

## Patterns of variation

Celts have a higher incidence of thoracic level NTD with severe cognitive deficit. Spaniards and Arabs have higher incidence of thoracic level NTD with severe hydrocephalus. Sikhs from Western Canada have higher incidence of thoracic level NTD with good motor function.

## Prenatal Diagnosis

Antenatal diagnosis of myelomeningocele has paved the way for modern treatment options in the form of *in utero* surgery and many other strategies in management of a child with myelomeningocele.

### Types of antenatal screening

There are two modalities of screening procedures offered to pregnant ladies in obstetric care. They include measuring maternal serum alpha-fetoprotein level and obstetric ultrasonography. If these two screening procedures come back positive then a more invasive test of amniocentesis is undertaken to confirm the diagnosis of MMCL. However, with the advent of advanced ultrasound resolution, measuring AFP has become less popular.

## AFP

In 1972, Brock and Sutcliffe were the first to establish a relationship between high alpha-fetoprotein level in amniotic fluids and open neural tube defect fetuses.

AFP is produced by fetal liver and yolk sac and is excreted in fetal urine into the amniotic fluid, from where it crosses the placental barrier and reaches maternal serum. Peak amniotic fluid AFP is found to be around 12 weeks. When the fetus has an open neural tube defect, AFP transudes from the exposed membrane into the amniotic fluid where its level starts to rise pathologically and this high level can move transplacentally and thus can be detected even in maternal serum. As it is an invasive procedure, amniocentesis is performed to measure the amniotic fluid AFP level only when a karyotype is needed to detect additional chromosomal anomalies in previously diagnosed pregnancies.

### Maternal AFP level

Maternal serum AFP is determined around second trimester of pregnancy between 15 and 22 weeks. The chosen cut-off value of 2.5 MoM (multiple of median) is considered positive. Women with AFP value greater than the cut-off limit should be referred for genetic counseling and consideration of diagnostic test in the form of targeted or level II ultrasound.

### Acetylcholine esterase

Acetylcholine is highly specific to neural tissue but is absent from the amniotic fluid. Thus its presence in the amniotic fluid is diagnostic of neural tube defect. Again, amniocentesis is undertaken only if karyotyping is necessary.

### Role of ultrasound in antenatal diagnosis
### of myelomeningocele

Traditional 2D ultrasound has replaced the maternal AFP measurement. While performing fetal ultrasound, gestational age has to be correlated with the ultrasound findings. There are two types of ultrasound examination offered to a pregnant lady as part of antenatal care. Screening ultrasound is undertaken in the second trimester by an obstetrician. If this screening ultrasound is positive for MMCL then the next step is to peform targeted or level II ultrasound. Targeted ultrasound is a specialized or advanced ultrasound for evaluation of the central nervous sytem along the spine. First trimester ultrasound is less sensitive for detecting MMCL as compared to second trimester ultrasound.

**Cranial signs**: There are three main sonographic cranial signs associated with myelomeningocele.

1. **"Banana sign"** represents the distorted cerebellum that has the shape of a banana due to the descend of the posterior fossa structures, the so-called Chiari type II malformation.
2. **"Lemon sign"**, refers to the shape of the skull seen in the transverse plane. It is caused by the concavity of the parietal bones. About 99% of children with spina bifida will have at least one of the above cranial findings at less than 24 weeks.
3. **Ventriculomegaly**, enlarged ventricles representing hydrocephalus.

**Spinal signs**: Presence of cystic lesion with splaying of posterior elements.

## Fetal Surgery

In developed countries, the concept of intrauterine repair of the myelo-meningocele has led to a multicenter study whose results will be declared shortly. Initally it was argued that the severity of damage to the exposed cord could be reduced through this early intervention. This original enthusiasm was supported by well-performed research studies in fetal sheep model for human MMCL. From these experimental studies it was observed that it is possible to preserve near normal leg movements after intrauterine repair.

The selection criteria for performing intrauterine repair is as follows:

1. The surgery had to be done before 26 weeks of gestation.
2. The fetus must have a normal karyotype, with absence of other congenital malformations.
3. Evidence of Chiari type II malformation present.
4. Absence of severe hydrocephalus (maximum lateral ventricular diameter <17 mm).
5. Normal leg movement *in utero* with absence of talipes foot or club foot deformity.
6. Lesion higher than sacral level 1.

The data collected in patients born after intrauterine repair of the MMCL defect was observed to have better preservation of movements of the lower extremities. However, eventually these children at a later age show the same degree of deficit in movement and ambulation as did the children who had undergone conventional repair of the defect.

On the other hand, it was observed that children who had intrauterine surgery did not develop Chiari type II as do their counterpart. The reason for this could be that by patching the leakage of CSF through the defect, the intraspinal pressure keeps the cerebellum within the confines of the posterior fossa.

It can be hypothesized that intrauterine surgery could facilitate the migration of periventricular neurons. Eventually this may prove beneficial for the architecture of the forebrain and reduce the incidence of epilepsy or prevent some cognitive deficits.

It has also been reported that children with lesions below L3 do become less shunt dependent. Certainly the risk for the life of the mother should not be overlooked when deciding if fetal surgery is an option.

## Delivery

In 1991, Cochrane *et al.* reported an ideal mode of delivery based on their finding on 208 children born with MMC. The authors concluded that there was no difference in the outcome of motor or sensory level on the basis of presentation, route of delivery, presence of labor or fetal distress. Only breech presentation was associated with higher incidence of wheelchair use with vaginal delivery, thus advocating Cesarean section for children born with breech presentation. Although the authors did caution that injury to the placode was inevitable in either of the cases with vaginal delivery or Cesarean section, the only relevant contradiction to vaginal delivery was the detection of the MMCL sac of more than 4 cm as the risk for rupture was higher.

However, it was Luthy *et al.* who advocated for Cesarean section as an ideal mode of delivery for children with MMCL with the intention that children with MMCL and with absence of hydrocephalus had a better outcome, especially if performed before the onset of labor. It is worth summarizing the essence of this study. The authors detected lesion on the

X-ray spine in the postnatal period, and defined the anatomical level which was considered to be the level of last intact vertebral lamina. This was then compared against the functional neurological level recorded at two years of age, and a numerical index was deduced. The anatomical level was numbered as cervical 1 to 8, thoracic 9 to 20, lumbar 21 to 25, sacral 26 to 29, and intact motor function 30. Sensory level was assessed by neurological and orthopedic examination and the level was determined and converted into the numerical score. The motor level was decided after examination of the child by a physical therapist. The final score was reported as the difference between initial score (anatomical and neurological) minus the final score (motor level). After such a thorough work the authors observed lower scores for children born via vaginal delivery as compared to children born via Cesarean section.

It is common to observe that there is loss of previously present lower limb movements during the first week in postnatal life. One of the possible mechanisms could be related to occurrence of spinal hemorrhages either as a result of secondary trauma incurred during vaginal delivery or from aberrant vessels which represent a spectrum of spinal dysraphism. This again favors Cesarean section as an ideal mode of delivery in such cases.

## Assessment of Newborn with Myelomeningocele

The neonatal assessment in a case of spina bifida is undertaken by keeping in mind the following concepts:

- Stabilization of the vitals
- Skin covered vs. non-skin covered defect. Is this a myelomeningocele? Answer to which leads determination of the modality of surgical intervention.
- Presence of any tears in the membrane (tears increases the risk of meningitis)
- Neurological level of defect
- Associated systemic involvement

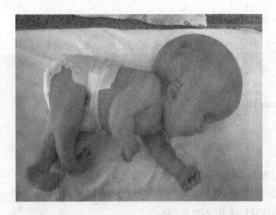

The child may have hydrocephalus, already clinically evident as the baby in the picture. In the above picture, the patient has enlarged scalp veins and tense fontanelle indicating hydrocephalus. The child has bilateral club feet, absence of plantar creases and with hip and knee in extended position, which is in concordance with his L2–L3 lesion. This increase of the intracranial pressure (normal range up to 5 mmHg in babies) may have caused brainstem compression and is manifested clinically by alterations in heart rate and blood pressure.

As an NTD is a congenital malformation, we have to search for other associated malformations such as:

- Cleft lip/cleft palate
- Anorectal anomalies like imperforate anus
- Associated congenital heart disease

## Cerebral function

- Look for level of alertness.
- Ability to fixate objects with eyes.
- Rule out hydrocephalus by palpating the anterior fontanelle.
- Look for dilated scalp veins. The child in the picture has dilated scalp veins.

## Cranial nerve assessment

- Look for strabismus/tongue fasciculation/presence of stridor/gagging reflex.

## Spinal cord function

*Motor*

- Look for spontaneous movements of legs.
- Assess the level from posture of legs (frog-like postures of legs indicate flaccid paralysis of lower legs).
- Assess spinal level from motor function.
- Look for any asymmetrical movement or posture of lower limbs (Table 1).

*Superficial reflexes*

- Look for anal wink.
- Stimulate the perianal region and look for anal sphincteric contraction which is indicative of functioning up to level S2 to S4.

## Bowel and bladder function

There are cases of lesions at S1 or S2. The attending physician would confirm that indeed the sphincters are not normal.

Table 1.   Muscle groups and nerves involved in movement of various joints.

| Joint | Movement | Muscle Groups | Nerves Involved |
| --- | --- | --- | --- |
| **Hip** | Flexion | Iliopsoas | Femoral nerve L1, L2, L3 |
| **Knee** | Flexion | Hamstrings | Sciatic nerve L4, L5, S1 |
| | Extension | Quadriceps | Femoral nerve L2, L3, L4 |
| **Ankle** | Dorsiflexion | Anterior tibialis | Anterior tibial nerve L4 and L5 |
| | Plantarflexion | Gastrocnemius and soleus | Sciatic nerve L5, S1, S2 |
| **Great toe** | Extension | Extensor hallucis longus | S1 |

- Presence of frequent, small volumes of dribbling of urine especially with crying, movement or suprapubic pressure is an indicator of future urinary incontinence.
- Patulous anus with constant leakage of meconium is also indicative of bowel incontinence.
- But in a note of hope, Stark *et al.* (1968) had made the following observations regarding bowel and bladder function.

  - Level of lower limb function is directly correlated with urological prognosis.
  - If lower limb function is normal then there will be an optimistic expectation with regards to the outcome of procedures aiming at restoring bladder and bowel continence.

## Orthopedic perspective

*Lower limb assessment*

- Ranges of passive movements at joints are assessed.
- At times there is no deformity present at birth but develops as the child grows.

## Diagnostic Investigations

- Cranial ultrasound — to rule out hydrocephalus. This test has the advantage of being simple, non-invasive and informative.
- MRI spine. Very often in the US and other developing nations we tend to disregard the value of an MRI, forgetting that there are other associated conditions, such as diastematomyelia that could be repaired at the time of the surgery. This associated conditions are not always evident at the time of the repair of the MMCL.
- CT/MRI brain. This is also for ruling out other malformations. I am of the idea that if the child has to go to the radiology suit we rather obtain an MRI of the brain and spine, just to decrease the exposure of the developing brain to radiation.

## Urodynamics

- Renal function test such as serum creatinine and serum urea
- Renal ultrasound and voiding cystourethrography (VCUG)

It is common to observe that there is loss of previously present lower limb movements during the first week in postnatal life. Although the exact mechanism for this early loss of motor function is not exactly known, the following is a description of possible etiologies:

The den Dunnen study from the Netherlands on histopathological features in autopsy findings from spina bifida-affected fetus which died from obstetric complications revealed the following points:

1. Reduced quantity of lower motor neurons
2. Aberrant spinal blood vessels
3. Occurrence of ependymal denudation

The inference drawn from the above study is that there is a pre-existing neural damage which is superimposed by additional damage to the cord during the process of delivery. From the pathological studies the neural damage was compatible with lower motor neuron type of damage.

The presence of spinal hemorrhages clearly indicate that either there is presence of aberrant blood vessels (from continuum of the neural tube defect process) or these hemorrhages are incurred during delivery process.

This study further supports the Cesarean section mode of delivery over the vaginal mode of delivery.

## Differential Diagnosis

The crux of the diagnosis of MMCL is the presence of a neural placode. In meningocele the skin of the sac or bulging mass is absolutely normal. In the case of a sacral teratoma this rare lesion is associated with the midline of the spinal canal in the neural placode.

Teratoma accounts for 3–9% of all spinal tumors. There have been reports of teratoma associated with myelomeningocele. Intra-operative finding of a sac that does not communicate with the spinal canal should raise suspicion for teratoma.

Hamartoma and human tail or appendage should also be considered, but considering that the appearance of the MMCL is so characteristic, rarely, if ever, a well-trained neonatologist will confuse it with any other lesion.

## Initial Preparations for Surgery

The exposed placode has to be covered with dura and skin. Until the OR is prepared the child has to remain prone with the myelomeningocele covered with a gauze embedded in sterile saline. A plastic wrap could be placed over the gauze to keep the placode moist. In any case what needs to be always kept in mind is that the placode is viable nervous tissue and it may still harbor sufficient neuronal structures to improve the general condition of the child. Thus what should never be done is to use any antiseptic solution over the placode.

## Surgery

It is advised that to prevent meningitis the MMCL must be closed ideally within the first day after birth. The great majority of patients with MMCL do not have other associated congenital conditions that would prevent a general anesthesia within 24 hours after birth.

If the child was born in a distant location and needs to be transferred to a tertiary center where surgery can be performed, the period for primary closure can be extended up to three days after birth. We recommend that the sac be punctured before surgery and the CSF evaluated at least for gross increase in cell number or for a Gram stain, particularly in cases when the child was transferred to the surgical center or when the time of the surgery has already passed 24 hours. Eventually the results provided by the CSF analysis could prove to be beneficial. In fairness I have to admit that I never had a positive culture.

Wide spectrum antibiotics are recommended for all cases. Precautions about latex allergy have to be maximized.

In the OR the child is positioned prone. The exposed area of the cord is not cleaned with antiseptics and is kept moist to prevent overheating from ceiling lights. The surgeon dissects the medullo vasculosa from the placode, followed by dissection of a plane of dura mater and suturing it over the placode. Some surgeons fold the placode restoring the tubular

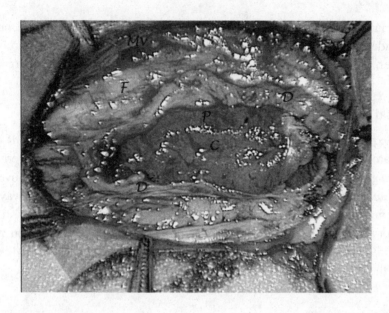

configuration of the cord, but there is no evidence that this affects the outcome of the surgery. The use of an artificial patch is also considered but there is no compelling evidence that it prevents tethering.

In the image above, the placode (P) with its central canal (C) has been detached from the skin and the dura mater (D) is already dissected in its entirety from the fascia (F) and will be sutured over the cord. The medullovasculosa (Mv) is being held by forceps; it will be removed before closing the skin.

All these efforts are evidence that after the defect has been properly closed, the golden standard that surgeons want to obtain is a mobile cord that will not delay the child's motor development by tethering. Some neurosurgeons prefer to engage a plastic surgeon to close the skin for defects that are larger than 5 centimeters in diameter.

The surgery usually lasts less than two hours. The child is placed on antibiotics for 24 hours. Ideally the child can be extubated at the end of the surgery but this decision is left to the anesthesiologist and the neonatologist. Simple steps like not holding the placode with a tooth or serrated forceps or just gentle utilization of suction and cauterization are enough.

After surgery the child has to rest prone, if possible but not obligatorily. The wound dressing has to be examined for evidence of CSF leakage. If present, the child needs to be shunted.

Unless there is severe malformation of the brain stem, the child should return extubated and can be fed orally in the coming hours.

## Delayed Surgery

The natural history of spina bifida cystica is unheard of in this modern era of medicine. In almost every corner of the developed world, primary treatment is initiated within a few hours after the delivery itself. In many countries surgeries are delayed because there is no immediate tertiary care for the child. Certainly, as discussed before, meningitis poses a significant threat to a child's life in cases where surgery is delayed.

The image below shows the presence of a sac which has epithelized and has rendered the child handicapped with limited level of motor function. Surgery will at least allow this particular child to have a better control of his trunk and help him in ambulation.

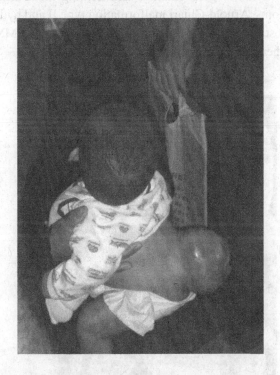

During preparation for surgery, the area over the placode is assumed to have been damaged by epithelization and thus in contrast with early surgery, the area is thoroughly cleaned with antiseptics. It has been observed that at four months, children with MMCL has a 51% chance of survival, and of those who reach one year, 77% will survive at least until they turn 12 years old. The cause of mortality varies according to age. In early stages, infection is the culprit, then hydrocephalus and finally, renal insufficiency.

## CNS Structures in Patients with MMCL

### Brain

The anatomical structure of the brain of patients with MMCL has been thoroughly studied with MRI. Those studies have unmasked a series of abnormalities that will be described below. Although we find a gamut of anomalies on radiological imaging, caution should be exercised in clinically correlating these radiological findings and treating them based on their clinical symptoms. Arnold-Chiari malformation type II and hydrocephalus are the two most important CNS pathologies accompanying MMCL. They are described here along with other anomalies.

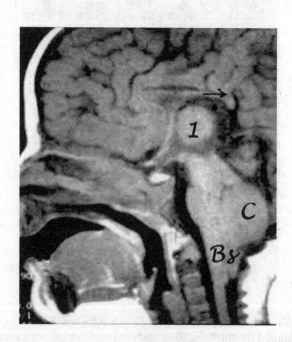

Some of the anomalies observed in the brain could be attributed to hydrocephalus and others seem to be independent of hydrocephalus and represent anomalies from the NTD itself.

Of the defects observed, the following are characteristics of MMCL:

1. *Thickened massa intermedia* (1). Interthalamic adhesions or enlarged massa intermedia corresponds to the medial aspect of the thalami across the third ventricle. These connections are not a true commisure due to absence of white matter fibers. Its significance is not yet determined other than the fact that it is associated with behavioral abnormalities like schizophrenia. The hypertrophy of the massa intermedia can be explained by either the small size of the third ventricle (secondary to CSF drainage or leak) or thalamic hypertrophy from overgrowth of the basal lamina, which belongs to the broader part of morphogenetic disturbances seen with spinal dysraphism. However, even children with normal cognitive development can have large massa intermedia as well.

2. The corpus callosum (arrow) and other commissures. Agenesis or dysplasia of corpus callosum is a common accompaniment especially of the posterior part of the commisure. However, a complete agenesis of corpus callosum has never been observed. The pathogenesis of the callosal defect is attributed to the broader aspect of global white matter defect seen to accompany these children. Although severe hydrocephalus is also known to be associated with white matter damage, the callosal dysplasia or agenesis seems to represent a true developmental anomaly. The aberrant crossing of cingulum fibers points towards yet another white matter dysplasia that cannot be explained by mere presence of hydrocephalus and thus favoring a true dysplasia in these children with MMCL and CM II. Another unusual feature noted with CM II is the dislocation of anterior commissural, which although unlikely, can represent an effect of hydrocephalus. It is not uncommon to find the septum pellucidum, corpus callosum and the fornix to be hypoplastic.

Thinning of the cerebral cortical mantle with selective posterior white matter thinning exceeding the anterior white matter thinning has been observed frequently in cases with CM II and MMCL. Modern technique that analyzes the white matter tracts with diffusion tensor imaging (DTI) suggests defective myelination. The etiology of the diffuse white matter dysplasia seen in children with CM II and MMCL can be attributed to the developmental anomaly with superadded effect of hydrocephalus.

*Neural Tube Defects*

## Skull and Osseous signs

1. Luckenschadel or lacunar skull
2. Scalloping of posterior surface of petrous pyramid
3. Enlarged foramen magnum

## Dural signs

1. Hypoplasia of falx cerebri
2. Fenestration of falx cerebri
3. Tentorial hypoplasia
4. Wide incisura

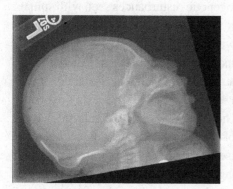 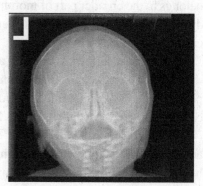

In the left image the flat occiput and lacunar skull can be observed. In the picture on the right, besides the lacunar skull, the diastased metopic suture, which is common in children with MMCL, can also be seen.

Luckenschadel skull, which means lacunar skull, is an almost forgotten entity which is commonly seen in Chiari type II malformation. With the advent of MRI and its widespread usage, CT or radiographic diagnosis of Chiari type II has been rendered obsolete. Nevertheless, the osseous pathologies observed in Chiari type II should not be undermined. On the contrary it should encourage readers to ponder on the pathophysiology of the primary defect in neural tube anomalies.

Luckenschadel or lacunar skull is always seen with myelomeningocele, meningocele and in encephalocele. In 85% of Chiari type II cases, lacunar skull is identified with ease.

As its name suggests, lacunar skull denotes presence of lacuna, meaning area of thinning, fenestrations or pits in the calvaria, especially noted in the frontal, parietal and the membranous occipital bone. It is detected on plain X-ray skull or CT scan with bone window. Both the inner and outer aspects of the skull are affected, especially seen with ease on the vertex, with brain tissue bulging into these pits.

In medical archives, reports of plain radiographs of pregnant ladies with myelomeningocele afflicted fetuses, presence of Luckenschadel deformity has been demonstrated. The lacunae may disappear in 1–2 months post-natally or may persist unchanged for a month or two. However, there is complete disappearance of these lacunae by six months of age in almost all cases, irrespective of the presence or absence of hydrocephalus.

## Petrous scalloping

In cases with Chiari type II on axial CT scans, flattening (10%) or frank concave scalloping (80%) of the petrous apex has been noted. The pressure from the growing cerebellum has been implicated for this bony erosion. Thus the frequency of finding the defect in the petrous bone increases with age. In fact the erosion is so obvious in older children that the scalloped margins of bilateral petrous pyramids form a single arc along with the scalloped posterior borders of the clivus. However, the petrous ridges and the jugular tubercles are spared from the erosion; [Kruyff and Jeffs].

## Enlarged foramen magnum

The foramen magnum is enlarged in 73% of cases with myelomeningocele. In radiographs it appears rounder than normal and with a small incisura in the region of opisthion (mid-point of the clivus).

## Hypoplasia of the falx cerebri

The anomalies of the falx include partial agenesis, hypoplasia or presence of fenestrations and are noted in 100% of cases with Chiari type II. The location of the anomaly may vary but the most commonly affected portions are the anterior and middle third of the falx.

This pathology is visualized in contrast-enhanced CT or in MRI. Fenestrations appear as gaps or focal interruption in the linear falx blush.

Secondary to falx hypoplasia, the cerebral hemispheres are closely apposed to each other with focal narrowing or obliteration of the intervening interhemispheric fissure; [Peach *et al.*].

## Tentorial hypoplasia

The tentorium cerebelli is hypoplastic in 95% of Chiari type II patients. The leaves of the tentorium are poorly developed, shallow and sickle-shaped. The resultant size of the posterior fossa is smaller than normal. This tentorial hypoplasia is well-visualized in contrast-enhanced CT.

## Wide incisura

As a result of maldevelopment of the tentorium cerebelli there is abnormal enlargement of the incisura especially in the sagittal plane.

## Spinal cord

The following characteristics are not obligatory but the possibility of associated lesions should never be underestimated by the medical team.

### Spinal cord cranial to the placode

1. Total or partial duplication of cord.
2. Hydromyelia or syringohydromyelia.
3. Presence of elongated canal.
4. Presence of arachnoid cyst.
5. Presence of surface fibrolipoma.
6. Presence of diplomyelia with duplicated central canal.
7. Presence of duplicated central canal without accompanying diplomyelia.
8. Absence of ventriculus terminalis.
9. Absence of organized cord tissue.

### Spinal cord at the level of placode

1. Flattened plate of neural tissue.
2. Necrosis of exposed dorsal surface.
3. Dorsal horn affected more than the ventral horns.
4. Local areas of syringomyelia.
5. Presence of complex mass of ependymal canals.

6. Various central canal anomalies such as slit-like central canal.
7. Massive necrosis throughout the plaque region.

## Histology of placode

1. Elongation of neural structures in the axial plane with a relative decrease in dorsal elements.
2. Paucity of number of neurons.
3. Presence of multiple areas of vacuolization and gliosis indicative of neural insult or injury.

## Histochemistry of placode

1. GFAP (glial cell marker) positivity throughout the placode except in areas of vacuolization.
2. Synaptophysin and chromogranin positive (neuronal marker).
3. HAM 56, a macrophage marker, is positive, indicative of severe inflammatory reaction.
4. Absence of peripheral neural markers in the placode but partially present in the peripheral elements.

## Neural placode at a glance (immunohistochemistry)

### 1. CD-44

CD-44 is an integral membrane glycoprotein and is a strong marker for ventral and periventricular or central caudal spinal cord with physiological absence in the junction between conus medullaris and filum terminale. In the MMCL placode this marker was present only in the ventral elements, yet again emphasizing the relative sparing of ventral elements as opposed to dorsal elements.

### 2. VIN-IS-53 and N-CAM

VIN-IS-53 is a monoclonal antibody that recognizes Neural Cell Adhesion Molecule (N-CAM). N-CAM is a group of glycoprotein present in neural crest cell derivatives and in the neural tube. Alterations in N-CAM are indicative of alterations in neurulation. Normally the VIN-IS-53 is strongly positive in the filum and can be seen faintly in the ventral conus which develop from secondary neurulation. In the MMCL placode there was strong staining at the ventral part of the placode. This very significantly shows the rostral pattern shift of the neural placode in MMCL.

## 3. AC4

AC4 is a specific marker for dorsal neural tube elements and is strongly positive for neuronal cell bodies and white matter in the normal human spinal cord. It is therefore positive for glial tissue.

## 4. FP3 and NOT1

FP3 and NOT1 are markers for glia and neuronal cell bodies of distal spinal cord. These markers are totally absent in MMCL placode, indicating the paucity of cell bodies in the placode. FP3 and NOT1 are markers for glia and neuronal cell bodies of distal spinal cord.

*Inference from histochemical study of myelomeningocele placode*

- Alterations of dorsoventral patterning and rostrocaudal patterning in the placode.
- Distortion of cord with relative sparing of the ventral elements.
- Presence of inflammatory and gliotic markers are indicative of secondary injury to the cord.
- Evidence of neural cell loss and spinal cord atrophy which may be due to injury or apoptosis or defective development.
- Alterations in developmental markers favor more towards developmental etiology for altered placode structure.

## Pathologies Associated with MMCL

### Hydrocephalus

In patients with MMCL, the CSF flow is blocked either at the level of the aqueduct of Sylvius by a congenital narrowing of the passage between the III and IV ventricles, or at the exit from the IV ventricles through the lateral foramen of Luschka and the median foramen of Magendie by the descended cerebellar tonsils that constitute an important part of the Chiari II complex.

When the newborn is lying supine and not crying, examination of the anterior fontanelle is a simple and fairly reliable method of gauging for intracranial pressure. If the fontanelle feels tense and is bulging over the edges of the suture then a bedside ultrasound, a head CT or brain MRI needs to be requested to further explore the meaning of this clinical sign and rule out hydrocephalus. Children with MMCL also have a gaping metopic suture that extends well into the middle of the forehead.

Usually at the time of birth, MMCL infants do not have overt signs of hydrocephalus as the CSF has leaked out through the spinal defect. This is observed even when the dorsal sac seems to be intact and filled with CSF.

For a while it was prevalent to place a ventriculoperitoneal shunt immediately after the closure of the MMCL, but this procedure has already been abandoned.

After the surgery, repeated head ultrasounds can give us an adequate estimate of the enlargement (if present) of the lateral ventricles. This together with assessment of the spinal wound will tell us if the CSF is under pressure in the cerebrospinal axis. Certainly, if the ventricles are not enlarged but there is evidence of CSF leak from the wound at the back, the patient definitely still needs to be shunted as CSF leak indicates high pressure.

As urological procedures, which will be discussed later, expose the peritoneal end of the shunt catheter to the environment, I consider such procedures to be a potential source of iatrogenic shunt infections. In general if the shunt was placed a year ago, I advice against taping the shunt for drawing CSF from the ventricle as this can also be a potential medium for shunt infection.

The figure below emphasizes that patients with MMCL are more prone to complications.

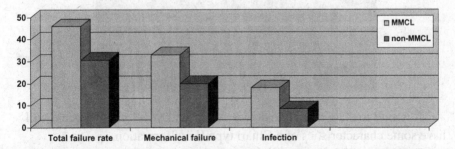

Fig. 2.   Bar graphs showing rates of total failure, mechanical failure and infection of MMCL patients as compared to non-MMCL patients.

## Chiari type II malformation

This clinical entity is named after Hans Chiari, a pathologist working in Prague, a territory of what was then the Austro-Hungarian Empire. In his works (around the time of 1891), on autopsy reports of cerebellar herniation syndromes, Chiari described the following significant criteria for diagnosis of CM II malformations: herniation of cerebellar vermis into the spinal canal below C2, with accompanying herniation of brain stem structures and fourth ventricle, and hydrocephalus. He also stated that this clinical entity of CM II is unique to MMCL children. There have been exceptions to this, especially in children who underwent intrauterine repair of the MMCL with no signs of Chiari II malformation, but nonetheless it is safe to assume that CM II always accompanies MMCL unless proven otherwise. The fact that symptomatic CM II is the most common cause of death in children with MMCL below two years of age, early recognition of its symptoms with prompt initiation of its management is advocated.

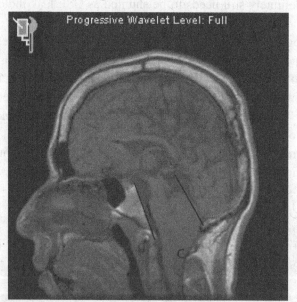

It is safe to state that almost every child with myelomeningocele will have some characteristics of a Chiari type II malformation.

The brain MRI shows the descent of the cerebellum (C), the brain stem and the vermis into the cervical canal. The posterior fossa is small;

this is evident by a tentorium running almost parallel to the clivus with a low insertion point. Two black lines run along the clivus at the left of the image and the tentorium at the right, indicating clearly the small volume of posterior fossa.

Two-thirds of the patients will evidence a dorsal "kink" of the medulla, if this is observed below C4, a great majority of the patients will have a distinctive propensity for Chiari II clinical manifestations, whereas when the kink is above C4 it does not have particular relation to outcome or prognosis.

## Pathogenesis of Chiari Malformation in MMCL

Out of the many theories forwarded to explain this condition, the one proposed by McLone and Knepper stands as the most plausible. It states that the constant drainage of CSF through the spinal defect induces the anatomical collapse of the ventricular system. The dilatation of the ventricular system acts as the scaffolding for the development of the calvarium, thus a small posterior fossa results from this collapsed ventricular system. This attractive theory has some indirect empirical confirmation. For one, children whose spinal defect was repaired *intra utero* do not develop Chiari as frequently as those treated after birth.

Years ago it was of common practice to place lumboperitoneal shunts for cases of pseudo-tumor cerebri and the indication was abandoned due to increased incidence of acquired Chiari. Both cases support the idea of an intact spinal fluid system needed to provide buoyancy to the cerebellum and prevent its descent.

There are two possible mechanisms of pathophysiology of Chiari II:

1. *Intrinsic brain stem malfunctions as a continuum of the MMC pathology.* In the literature it is reported that younger children become symptomatic in a severely progressive and rapid manner and are less likely to improve with decompressive surgery, raising the possibility of intrinsic brain stem defect.
2. *Brain stem/cervical cord compression.* The symptoms develop later in life. As decompression is helpful in relieving them we conclude that the symptoms were related to compression. In my opinion, the so-called compression is related to increased intracranial pressure secondary to a

poorly functioning shunt. When the surgeon opens the dura mater, this relieves the CSF pressure and expands the diameter of the cord through laminectomy thus pressure of the system is reduced.

## Clinical presentations of Chiari type II

Brain stem dysfunction, more commonly observed in infants.

- Feeding and swallowing difficulties
- Neurogenic dysphagia
- Poor feeding and palatal weakness
- Gastroesophageal reflux and aspiration pneumonia
- Visual disturbances and diplopia

Upper and lower respiratory pathologies:

- Vocal cord paralysis and weak or low pitched cry
- Prolonged breath holding spell
- Central apnea

Spinal cord dysfunction, more commonly observed in older children.

- Unsteady gait
- Incoordination of movements
- Nystagmus
- Truncal ataxia
- Appendicular ataxia

## Common GI complaints in children with myelomeningocele

In children with myelomeningocele, GI complaint predominates with presence of one of the following symptoms:

- Swallowing difficulty
- Vomiting
- Poor feeding
- Episodes of choking, coughing and wheezing during feeding
- Nasal regurgitation of food
- Failure to thrive

The abovementioned symptoms vary with age. It is the mother who usually complains that her child has spells of coughing, choking and wheezing whenever she feeds her baby. Either forceful vomiting without precedent nausea or even in some cases spitting is a common complaint seen in these children. At the most extreme end of the spectrum the child cannot tolerate oral feeds at all and this results in failure to gain weight and thus *failure to thrive*.

### Child below two years of age

*Respiratory system*: The most common and perhaps the most lethal of symptoms to evolve are pertinent to the respiratory system and clinically they manifest as shortness of breath and stridor, mostly in the form of inspiratory stridor, pathological loss of protective reflexes resulting in aspiration and choking, followed by frequent chest infections. The pediatrician plays an imperative role of recognizing these early signs and also differentiating them from common viral upper respiratory infections in this age group. On examination the child with a laryngoscope, vocal cord abduction paresis or paralysis is noted, which confirms the diagnosis. The most extreme form of respiratory pathology that can affect is in the form of apnea where there is total cessation of expiratory effort with resultant cyanosis, leading to bradycardia and even to death. These lethal events can be triggered by startling and can even occur in mechanically ventilated cases. This apneic spells in children with MMCL should never be confused with breath holding spells commonly seen in the same age group and should be managed immediately in the form of posterior fossa decompression. Along with accompanying apnea of central origin, there are a gamut of sleep-disordered breathing arising mostly from palatal weakness and subsequently complex surgical procedures such as uvulopharyngopalatoplasty are needed.

*Gastrointestinal symptoms*: The gastrointestinal symptoms are more insidious in origin and are clinically manifested as neurogenic dysphagia presenting with feeding and swallowing difficulties, recurrent aspiration, choking and vomiting, nasal regurgitation, prolonged feeding time and weight loss even to the extent of failure to thrive. On physical examination of such cases, absence of gag reflex, coarse upper respiratory sounds and emaciation will be noted as positive findings. Barium swallow and other studies of the upper gastrointestinal tract may show pharyngoesophageal dysmotility, cricopharyngeal achalasia, nasal regurgitation and even frank tracheal aspiration.

*Other systemic complaints*: Other symptoms attributed to CM II are upper limb weakness, hypotonia, sleep-disordered breathing, and opisthotonus.

### Approach to swallowing dysfunction in a child with myelomeningocele

Neurogenic dysphagia is defined as a functional disorder characterized by difficulty in swallowing due to abnormal neural control of the swallowing process leading to incoordinate propulsion and peristalsis of the food bolus.

### Causes of neurogenic dysphagia in myelomeningocele

- Stretching of cranial nerves by the caudal displacement of medulla.
- Intrinsic dysgenesis of cranial nerve nuclei in the brain stem.

### Diagnostic investigations

Whenever a child with myelomeningocele presents with any complaint related to feeding intolerance, they should be subjected to formal swallowing studies which include the following:

- Cine-esophagogram (peristalsis)
- Manometry studies (achalasia)
- 24-hour pH monitoring (to detect presence of reflux)
- Radionuclide scintigraphy or milk scans (to detect aspiration in lungs)

### Respiratory complaints in children with myelomeningocele

Children born with myelomeningocele are at increased risk of cardio-respiratory failure from lower brain stem dysfunction. The following are common types of respiratory complaints observed in children with myelomeningocele and Chiari II.

- Central sleep apnea and other disturbance in central respiratory control
- Upper airway dysfunction
- Vocal cord palsy and stridor

- Aspiration pneumonia
- Cor pulmonale

The respiratory dysfunction seen in myelomeningocele with Chiari type II will be explained in this section. For the sake of description we will divide the respiratory dysfunction into upper airway and lower airway dysfunction.

*Upper airway dysfunction*

- Sleep apnea
- Sleep disordered breathing

*Lower airway dysfunction*

- Vocal cord paralysis
- Loss of protective cough reflex
- Aspiration
- Inspiratory stridor
- Anesthetic implications

Common clinical complaints presented by mother of the child with myelomeningocele and Chiari type II are described here. The complaints in infancy pertain mainly to severe lower airway dysfunction and has an early onset as compared to older children who present with upper airway disorder. The following are common complaints mentioned:

- Weak cry
- Noisy breathing
- Choking and coughing during feeds
- Breathing difficulty

Upper airway signs manifest at a later age with the following types of complaints:

- Breathing difficulty during sleep
- Snoring with episodes of apnea
- Daytime somnolence and headaches

The pathophysiologies behind these respiratory symptoms have a combined central and peripheral dysfunction of control of respiration. A short summary of the physiological control of rate and rhythm of respiration is mentioned here. To begin with this discussion, we will first explain the upper airway mechanics followed by factors influencing the lower airways.

*Upper respiratory tract*

Upper respiratory tract is defined as the area starting from the posterior nasal septum to the inlet of the larynx which is guarded by the epiglottis. As there is no bony support for the upper airway, it has a natural tendency to collapse.

The following are two important mechanisms by which the upper airways remain patent:

i. *Role of pharyngeal dilators*
Genioglossus and tensor veli palatini are two important muscles that are primary forces opposing the collapse of the upper airways. The genioglossus is supplied by the XII nerve while the tensor veli palatini is supplied by the V3 (mandibular nerve V).

The genioglossus is a phasic muscle, which means that it is activated during inspiration and less activated during expiration, as opposed to tensor veli palatini, which is a tonic muscle which remains activated with the same intensity throughout the respiratory cycle.

ii. *Longitudinal traction of the upper airways by lung inflation during inspiration*
During inspiration, the lungs expand and this creates a negative intraluminal pressure which activates the pharyngeal dilators. The net result is longitudinal traction of pharynx with opposing forces that tend to collapse the airways.

*Central control of upper airways*

i. **Primary signals**
*Sensors or receptors*: There are mechanoreceptors present in the walls of upper airways that detect negative pressure.
*Input*: The signals from these receptors are carried to the medullary respiratory center by the superior laryngeal branch of the vagus X nerve.
*Control center*: The medullary respiratory center sends signals to the hypoglossal motor nucleus, i.e. the XII nerve.

*Output*: The efferent signal to the genioglossus muscle is carried by the XII nerve or the hypoglossal nerve.

ii. **Secondary signals**

Following are the types of inputs to the hypoglossal motor nuclei (XII) which also leads to activation or contraction of the pharyngeal dilators.

- Medullary respiratory neurons during the inspiration phase
- Serotonergic and noradrenergic signals from the medullary center involved with awake/asleep state

*Key notes*

*Awake state*:

Upper airways patent due to

1. Activation of pharyngeal dilators (the most important factor)
2. Development of negative intraluminal pressure from lung inflation
3. Positive respiratory drive from awake state (serotonin/noradrenalin)

*Pathology of upper airway dysfunction in myelomeningocele children*

- Sleep disorder breathing
- Sleep apnea

*Explaining sleep apnea*

Sleep apnea seen in Chiari patients are a combination of central sleep apnea and obstructive sleep apnea with a dominance of obstructive pattern.

*Mechanism*

The following are two possible theories to explain sleep apnea in children with myelomeningocele.

i. *Depression of respiratory drive*

Compression of medullary respiratory system by the herniated cerebellum decreases the ventilatory drive. This leads to hypoventilation and collapsing of the upper airways.

ii. *Chemoreceptor dysfunction*

Either abnormal sensitivity of the peripheral chemoreceptor to hypoxia or abnormal processing of the input from these receptors can lead to sleep apnea. The reason could be due to either stretching of the lower cranial nerves or brain stem dysfunction.

The symptoms mentioned above are related to the structural anomalies of the posterior fossa. But why they have chosen to manifest well after birth is an unsolved puzzle.

There is more or less a consensus among pediatric neurosurgeons towards considering shunt revision even though there is no clear radiological evidence of enlargement of ventricles. Any form of cognitive, motor or sensory dysfunction of the child can possibly mean shunt malfunction. Impaired handwriting, irritability, and upper hand weakness are to be seriously evaluated even if there is no evidence of shunt failure and the MRI shows what we already knew since the child was born; that he has a Chiari II malformation.

## Treatment

In an infant with stridor or any other form of respiratory distress, e.g. secondary to frequent bouts of pneumonia, the shunt has to be revised. If the symptoms do not subside then it should proceed with a cervical laminectomy. As the foramen magnum is already enlarged there is no point in performing a suboccipital craniectomy as in Chiari I. Nonetheless the edges of the foramen magnum can be removed no more than one centimeter from its original level. This is advised to facilitate the incision and, more importantly, during closure of the dura.

The cerebellar tonsils should never be tampered with. The tonsils are adhered to the brain stem and significant damage can result when the surgeon searches for a plane between them. Excessive cervical laminectomy can cause spine instability.

In an older child the same principle applies. But in my experience the revision of the shunt, even if the ventricles are not enlarged in consecutive head CT or brain MRI, usually alleviates the symptoms.

## Latex allergy

Children with myelomeningocele have been found to have allergic reactions to latex and latex products. Repeated surgical procedures, catheterizations and placement of implants containing latex have been implicated as the explanation for the presence of latex allergy. Incidence of latex allergy in spina bifida children is 29–64%.

Allergy to latex products falls under type I allergic reactions which are mediated by IgE antibodies and is an immediate type of reaction. In children with myelomeningocele there are two distinct conditions, namely latex allergy and latex sensitizations. Latex sensitization is presence of IgE reaction against latex products but the children are asymptomatic as compared to children with latex allergy who have clinical manifestations. Yet the first group of children is vulnerable to serious latex allergy.

*Clinical picture of latex allergy*

Clinically, latex allergy can manifest as one of the following conditions:

- Urticaria
- Angioedema
- Rhinitis
- Conjunctivitis
- Asthma
- Generalized anaphylactic reaction

As is evident from the abovementioned conditions, the clinical picture of latex allergy can be variable. It can range from minor skin hives or urticaria to the most severe anaphylactic reactions, although serious allergic reactions are more commonly seen after mucosal exposure.

Appearance of any of the clinical features mentioned below should alert the treating physician of possible allergic reaction to latex.

**Urticaria:** The appearance of erythematous, itchy, circular, blanchable papules of size 1 to 2 cm constitutes urticaria. Urticaria usually remains discrete or may coalesce and involves the superficial dermis.

**Angioedema:** The involvement of deeper dermis or tissues by edema is called angioedema. Usually urticaria and angioedema are seen as a spectrum of the same pathology.

**Allergic rhinitis:** Immediately after exposure to the allergen such as latex, the appearance of repeated bouts of sneezing followed by itching of eyes and nose associated with clear rhinorrhea or nasal congestion is diagnostic of allergic rhinitis.

**Allergic conjunctivitis:** The onset of itching and watering of eyes with associated redness of eyes is a sign of allergic conjunctivitis and is usually seen with allergic rhinitis. There is complete absence of any purulent discharge from the eyes.

*Management of latex allergy reactions*

Use of H1 antihistaminics like diphenhydramine or Benadryl is recommended. For older children the non-sedating antihistaminics like cetirizine or loratadine can be used.

**Asthma**

Immediately after exposure to latex, if the child starts to cough with associated presence of wheezing, the physician should be alerted. Presence of dyspnea and increasing effort of breathing should alert the physician to start prompt treatment in the form of inhalation of B2 agonist like albuterol or terbutaline puffs.

**Anaphylaxis**

Anaphylaxis is the most severe and life threatening clinical condition with hemodynamic compromise in the form of hypotension, wheezing and respiratory obstruction from laryngeal and pharyngeal edema with severe dysnea, urticaria and angioedema. Immediate administration of subcutaneous or intramuscular adrenaline of 1 in 1000 units is life-saving treatment. The dose may be repeated in 15 to 20 mins. Management further includes administration of hydrocortisone, antihistaminic, inhalation of B2 agonist and maintaining hydration.

*Pathogenesis of latex allergy in spina bifida patients*

The propensity of latex mediated allergic reaction seen in MMCL is considered an intrinsic defect of MMCL and the effect of multiple exposures to latex products causing allergic reactions is secondary and not the main pathology. This fact can be explained by comparison with control groups, for instance, in infants with post-hemorrhagic hydrocephalus undergoing shunt placement and with comparable exposure to latex products. Yet in these children there is a much lower rate of latex allergy.

Early contact of meninges with latex powder which subsequently leads to an atopic immune response seems like a possible explanation for the high incidence of latex allergy in children with MMCL.

Rubber particles are water insoluble and thus cannot transfer from gloves to skin of healthcare workers, but they can transfer to mucosal membranes of body cavities like meninges.

## Endocrine

Midline central nervous system disorders like septo-optic dysplasia, dysgenesis of corpus callosum and basal encephalocele are known to be accompanied by abnormalities of hypothalamic–pituitary axis. MMCL is also included in this group and is known to be associated with endocrine issues mainly in the form of short stature and central precocious puberty, which are the two most prevalent hormonal disturbances seen in MMCL children.

### Short stature

It has been universally reported that the lower the lesion, the greater the normalcy in height and vice versa. For instance, S1 and lower level of defect was noted to have acquired height within the normal range. The mean height acquired by MMCL children are 141 cm for women and 152 cm for men, which is way smaller than the normal height range of their peers in the same age group. Researchers also found low total body potassium which decreased with age and this represented decrease primarily in lean body mass. The following are various possible etiologies of short stature in children with MMCL. The author agrees on dividing the etiologies into those which are modifiable into those which not modifiable (meaning those which cannot be averted even by proper treatment).

Modifiable etiologies of short stature in MMCL:

- Hydrocephalus
- Infections which tend to be recurrent and chronic
- Nutritional problems
- Contractures
- Renal disease (this can be prevented by regular urological follow up)

Non-modifiable etiologies for short stature in MMCL:

- Level of lesion
- Scoliosis, kyphosis and lordosis along with other vertebral bony anomalies
- Neurotrophic effect like precocious puberty
- Lower limb and trunk hypoplasia
- Hydrocephalus and tethered cord syndrome

*Precocious puberty*

- **Definition:** Precocious puberty is defined as onset of pubertal features like thelarche before nine years of age.
- **Possible causes are:** Hydrocephalus, especially raised intracranial pressure during perinatal period.
- **Incidence:** 6–11%
- **Treatment:** GnRH analogs such as Lupron. (Side effects of Lupron include osteoporosis and hot flushes.)

## Respiratory

There is a compromise in the respiratory muscle function in children with myelomeningocele especially those with upper lesion (cervicothoracic).

| Groups | PiMax (Maximum Inspiratory Pressure) cm $H_2O$ | PeMax (Maximum Expiratory Pressure) cm $H_2O$ |
|---|---|---|
| Control | 83 | 87.4 |
| Myelomeningocele (cervicothoracic) | 38.3 | 48 |
| Myelomeningocele (lumbosacral) | 60.8 | 71.7 |

## Neuro-opthalmology

Less than 5% of children with MMC have visual field defects on formal visual field charting. Opthalmic origin of headache should be in the differentials of headache in children with myelomeningocele.

Children with myelomeningocele have in more than 90% of cases associated with Chiari malformation, characterized by caudal displacement of cerebellum and the lower brain stem. These pathologies along with presence of raised intracranial pressure may contribute to ocular disturbances seen commonly in these children and may affect quality of life.

The various types of ocular disturbances seen in children with myelomeningocele are:

i. Visual perception, which includes:
   - Visual acuity
   - Refractive errors
   - Accommodation
   - Color vision

ii. Defective extraocular muscle movements
   - Strabismus
   - Nystagmus

iii. Optic atrophy

i. *Visual perception*

- **Visual acuity**
  MMC children have delayed visual acuity maturation which is noted from various studies mentioned in the literature. At the age of 12–14, almost 71% of children had normal visual acuity which they did not have at a younger age.

- **Refractory errors**
  From most of the studies, an incidence of 55–81% of refractive errors has been reported in children with myelomeningocele. A short explanation of different types of refractive errors is described here.
  *Astigmatism*:
  This is the most common type of refractive error seen in children with myelomeningocele. Astigmatism is defined as a defect where there are two planes of focus arising when either the cornea or the lens is not completely spherical.

  Early correction is necessary otherwise it will cause decrease in vision called *amblyopia*. Usually astigmatism coexists with hypermetropia or far-sightedness, which is explained as when the child cannot see near objects but retains distant vision.

Large uncorrected hyperopia can cause strabismus (esotropia) concurrent with amblyopia. The normal process of emmetropization which includes decrease in physiological astigmatism does not take place in these children. Thus astigmatism combined with hypermetropia is the predominant refractive error noted in these children.

- **Accommodation**
  Defective neural control may result in poor accommodation sometimes with normal visual acuity.
- **Color vision**
  There is mention of very few studies with decreased red-green color vision.

ii. *Defective extraocular movements*

- **Strabismus**
  Strabismus is defined as malalignment of the two visual axes. An incidence of 40–50% of strabismus is seen in children with MMCL, with the most common form of strabismus being esotropia versus exotropia, which is rarely seen in children with MMCL.

  Early treatment of strabismus or squint eye is necessary for development of full visual potential. Apart from the medical aspects, strabismus can have a social implication.

  There are two basic types of strabismus, namely esotropia and exotropia.

*Esotropia*

This is defined as excessive convergence of the visual axes. Esotropia can also be secondary to uncorrected large degree of hyperopia or farsightedness. Surgery is the mainstay of treatment in these cases.

*Exotropia*

Excessive divergence of visual axes of the two eyes is called exotropia and is usually secondary to neurological conditions like lacteral rectus palsy seen in hydrocephalus cases. As with effective control of hydrocephalus, this type of strabismus is rarely encountered in the present clinical settings.

Etiology of strabismus

1. Presence of hydrocephalus is associated with lateral rectus palsy innervated by the 6th nerve.
2. Intrinsic lesions of cerebellum and the brain stem may lead to various ocular motility defects, including weakness of oblique muscles which result in A and V pattern of deficits.

- **Nystagmus**
  Nystagmus is defined as rhythmic oscillations of the eye. "Side-pocket" type of nystagmus is a form of nystagmus that is described as the most common form of nystagmus seen in children with MMCL and Chiari type II. Recently a correlation between degree of tectal beaking and the severity of nystagmus has been defined.

iii.   *Optic atrophy*

With modern treatment strategy to control and treat hydrocephalus, the incidence of this entity of optic atrophy has been markedly decreased.

**Neurocognitive**

*Neuropsychological profile of children with spina bifida*

Neurocognitive development in children with myelomeningocele displays a dynamic pattern and is adversely affected by multiple factors such as neurological abnormalities, medical conditions and their interventions, as well as environmental challenges.

Serial neuropsychological test can assess damage and at the same time differentiate deficits due to intrinsic abnormal pathological continuum of MMCL from those deficits incurred due to medical conditions such as hydrocephalus and Chiari type II.

Children with MMCL have displayed consistent impairment in executive functions mainly restricted to frontostriatal connections throughout the treatment course but have shown improvement in other areas of neurocognitive profile during periods of medical stability.

*Pathophysiology*

- Executive functions depend on integrity of connections between frontal lobes and cerebellum/thalamus/striatum.
- Cerebellum plays an important role in skillful learning and automatization which prevents overlearning and habitualization like in learning handwriting.
- With cerebellar dysfunction, the child has more effortful and time-consuming cognitive processing, leading to slower and imperfect task performance.
- This can secondarily lead to the child feeling frustrated, fatigue and forgetful, subsequently affecting learning and executive functions.

*Neuropsychological domains of interest*

i. *Attention skill performance*

   The Conners' Continuous Performance Test (CPT) reported that shunt revision results in major improvement on certain areas of the CPT test, including omission error, response time and variability. However, there was no change in commission errors which indicate inhibitory control.

ii. *Verbal memory*

   The Wide Range Assessment Memory and Learning Test called WRAML by Adams and Sheslow was used. Memory scores were poor during periods preceding shunt malfunctions and remained baseline with revisions but improved significantly during stable medical periods. On the other hand, poor scores were persistent in Learning and Delayed Recall Trial scoring systems. The test used with the purpose of detecting these areas of memory is California Verbal List Learning task — the children's version is called CVLT-C; [Delis *et al.*]. Poor performance on this test remained even during periods of medical stability. This shows that executive functions which require more mental effort like recall memory using clues instead of recall memory with simple recognition, is abnormal in children with MMCL.

iii. *Visual perception*

   Visual-spatial and visual-perceptual skills together account for Visual Perception Task. Visual-spatial ability is dictated by Judgment of Line Orientation test and Visual Perception Test is dictated by Beery Test.

Improvement in both these tests have been noted after shunt revisions, clearly indicating the damaging effects of hydrocephalus have on the development of these mental faculties.

iv. *Visual memory*

Visual memory is tested with the following battery of tests which include:

1. Rey–Osterrieth Complex Figure Test (ROCF)
2. Developmental Scoring System
3. Children's Memory Scale
4. Dot locations and faces subset

Poor results were obtained consistently across all the tests with improvement in the post-operative period. The ability to correctly answer "where" tests the dorsal/parietal visual system and the "what" tests the ventral/temporal visual system.

v. *Visual motor skills*

The impact of hydrocephalus is clearly seen in the improvement of visual motor integrative skills after shunt revisions. However, consistent impairment in dexterity of manual functions is seen even after shunt revisions.

vi. *Adaptive skills*

Variable results have been obtained although the testing results are subjective in nature. Some environmental and social influences are involved here.

*Summary of neuropsychological studies*

- The following skills did not show any improvement with shunt revisions or stable medical conditions:

  1. Inhibitory control (commission errors)
  2. Organization
  3. Spontaneous verbal knowledge
  4. Retrieval skills

- This persistent deficit indicates that executive functions are impaired in children with MMCL.
- Impact of hydrocephalus on certain areas of executive functions is clearly seen with improving visuomotor integrational skills (VMI) after

shunt revisions. Visuomotor integration is related to visuoconstructive complexity.

- However, these patients lacked the visuoconstructional and organizational skills applied simultaneously and immediately, which places higher demands on executive function, showing yet another example of impaired executive ability.
- Recall of location "where" over faces "what" indicate a preferential sparing of spatial visual memory over object visual memory.

## Conclusion

Obstructive hydrocephalus has selective effects on long-term neurobehavioral functions most commonly affecting executive functions. With the advances in neurosurgical treatment modalities, the neurocognitive development in children with myelomeningocele has improved dramatically. However, it has been reported recently that although children with MMCL have IQ within the normal range, the IQ is on the lower end of the range. Approximate range of IQ in children with MMCL is 96.62 with a variation of 13 units, which is not considered retarded by DSM-IV classification. IQ depends on multiple factors which include interplay with genetic and environmental factors.

The following are possible causes of low performance in IQ testing for children with MMCL:

- Anomalous cerebral and cerebellar development as an intrinsic defect in MMCL.
- Raised intracranial pressure or inadequately treated hydrocephalus. In fact, presence of hydrocephalus lowers the IQ by 10% as compared to the general population.

The following are inferred from radiological images seen in children with MMCL and lower IQ levels:

- Anomalous development of corpus callosum especially the splenium.
- Tectal beaking.
- Deficient gray and white matter development in the cerebral cortex.
- Deficient development of neocerebellum or the lateral cerebellar hemisphere.

*Explaining IQ performance in children with MMCL*

There is a definite difference of IQ levels between MMCL children with high level of defect and those with low level of defect. By low level defect we are referring to the lumbosacral MMCL which is also the commonest of defects, in comparison with the high level of defect which is the thoracic level of MMCL.

From pathological study of children who died with thoracic level MMCL, the thickness of the cortical mantle was observed to be markedly less than those with lumbosacral level. The incidence of anomalous brain development such as agenesis of the corpus callosum was also found to be higher in children with high levels of MMCL. Considering the complicated perinatal course and difficulty nursing children with thoracic level of MMCL, it is also well accepted that children with thoracic level MMCL have poorer outcome compared to lower MMCL.

*Results of IQ testing in children with MMCL: possible role of ethnicity*

Most children with MMCL have not only lower range of IQ but also have deficits in higher cognitive functions such as poor memory and retrieval abilities associated with impaired executive functions. Upper levels of MMCL are associated with greater deficits in intellectual, academic and adaptive behavior. Mixed handedness is also seen commonly with high levels of defects.

Children born to Hispanic mothers have greater incidence of pervasive impairment of intellectual functions. Possible role of socioeconomic status has been noted. Children born to non-Hispanic mothers have lower MMCL level and greater verbal IQ and stronger adaptive behavior in social communication skills.

*Neurocognitive phenotype in children with MMCL*

Children with MMCL have the following common deficits:

1. Timing of processing information
2. Attention orientation
3. Motor learning

**1. Timing of processing information**
   Anomalous development of neocerebellum or the lateral cerebellar hemispheres can explain the slow processing of information seen

in children with MMCL. The fine motor control and coordination of movements are impaired in these children, as seen in impaired handwriting skills in children with MMCL.

2. **Attention orientation**

   Anomalous mid-brain development is associated with impaired eye movement coupled with shifting attention which accounts for the impaired attention oriented learning.

3. **Motor learning**

   Core deficits in motor learning arise from impairment of two processes, namely assembled processing and associated processing of information. Children with MMCL have intact associated processing (ability to recall events without intention of remembering) as compared to impaired attentive processing (conscious effort to store and recall). Perceptual difficulties are related to posterior cortex thinning.

*Why IQ is not an ideal indicator of cognitive functions in children with MMCL?*

Children with MMCL fail to acquire age-appropriate cognitive skills even in the absence of shunt malfunction.

   Under these conditions, sole IQ testing has poor predictive validity and on the contrary may lead to overestimating independent functioning in children with MMCL due to impaired motor and executive functioning in these children.

## Orthopedic

Orthopedic issues are addressed as a part of multidisciplinary treatment approach to children with myelomeningocele. The following are description of orthopedic pathologies seen in these children.

### Hip dislocation

One of the commonest pathologies seen in children with myelomeningocele is spontaneous hip dislocation. This pathology is classically observed with lower lumbar level of namely L3–L4 level myelomeningocele and arises due to asymmetry of muscle action. However, hip dislocation can be seen with neurological deficit at any level and not necessarily lead to significant impairment of ambulatory function. As the hips are dislocated over a period of time, there is absence of accompanying pain. This supports the conservative management of hip dislocation unless there is development of flexion contractures which necessitates operative procedure to release the contractures.

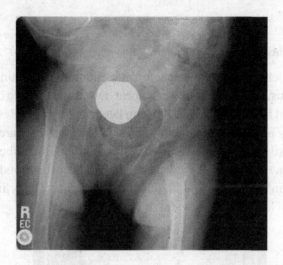

The only exception where hip dislocation needs more proactive treatment approach is the presence of unilateral hip dislocation associated with low level MMCL, raising the possibility of tethered cord.

## Knee contractures

Knee contractures are sequela of two interrelated conditions: tethered cord syndrome or true flexion contractures, which again might arise from tethered cord syndrome or asymmetric strength in the hamstrings. The hamstrings which include muscles semitendinosus, semimembranosus and biceps femoris are the main flexors of the knee joint and are innervated by the tibialis branch of sciatic nerve corresponding to spinal level L3, L4 and L5. The result of knee contractures is a crouching stance and gait, subsequently leading to impairment of ambulation. The classical picture includes tendon and intracapsular contractures, depending on previous ambulatory status. If the child was ambulated before, then flexion contractures as low as 20° warrants active management. On the other hand, if the child was wheelchair bound then larger degrees of contractures as high as 90° can be tolerated before the child complains of pain.

Treatment consists of release with tenotomy combined with capsulec-tomy with release of intra-articular structures. Before proceeding with an orthopedic procedure, the possibility of tethered cord should be ruled out first as mild degrees of deformity may halt or even revert to untethering procedure.

## Foot deformities

Foot deformities are a common accompaniment of myelomeningocele and include equinus, equinovarus and calcaneal deformities. These deformities may be present from birth or may develop later right up to adolescence age. The pathology behind development of these foot deformities are either due to tethered cord syndrome or syringomyelia and they should be addressed first before any orthopedic procedures. It has been observed that mild deformities can be reversible with untethering of cord. Delay in initiating treatment may lead to development of contractures.

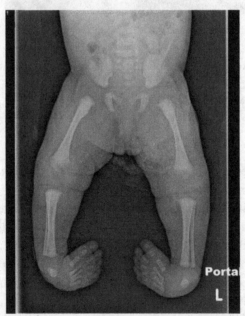

The initial management consists of stretching and casting, especially performed in calcaneal deformity cases. Clubfoot, or *talipes equinovarus*, can be managed as above with the Ponseti brace, but the process is very lengthy and might interfere with compliance to treatment. The only complication of this bracing or casting method is the development of pressure sores.

Surgical procedures include release of Achilles tendon or the anterior tibial tendon. After the release of tendons, the foot is supported by orthotics and braces which will maintain the foot in position and not lead to pressure sores.

### Spine deformities

Spine deformities can arise from either congenital vertebral anomalies or from progressive neurological changes from presence of tethered cord syndrome or syringomyelia. The most common spinal deformities seen in these children are scoliosis and kyphosis.

**Scoliosis**: Defined as lateral spinal curvature in the frontal plane and is diagnosed accurately on the anteroposterior view of an X-ray spine. Curvature may be single or multiple and are always described in the direction of the convexity. Scoliosis can arise from congenital deformities of the vertebral column like hemivertebra or butterfly vertebra, or from secondary pathologies of the spinal cord such as syringomyelia, tethered cord syndrome or shunt failure. In either case scoliosis leads to significant deformity and impairment of ambulation.

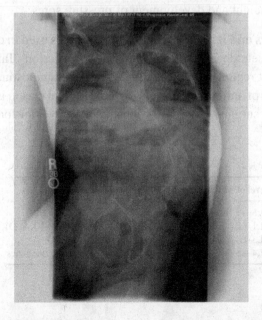

*Neural Tube Defects*

The image above also shows bladder calculi, a known condition in patients with MMCL.

Before undertaking any orthopedic correction of scoliosis, the spinal pathologies mentioned above should be ruled out first. A clue to underlying spinal pathology consists of presence of progressive scoliosis which usually indicates presence of syrinx or tethered cord. Untethering has led to improvement in the above conditions.

Orthopedic treatment is in the form of bracing or fusion surgeries. However, bracing and application of orthotics not necessarily halt the progression of curve but helps buy time for skeletal maturity. This is also in light of the fact that these children with underlying myelopathy with decreased sensation are prone to development of pressure sores.

**Kyphosis**: Defined as forward bending or hyperflexion of the spine in the sagittal plane. It is best detected from the lateral view of an X-ray spine.

Kyphosis is a more serious condition as compared to scoliosis. This spinal deformity usually accompanies higher level myelomeningocele defects such as high lumbar or thoracic level and is progressive in nature.

Kyphotic deformity is present from birth and arises from congenital vertebral deformity such as hemivertebra or as a result of segmentation failure. Any delay in initiating treatment can have serious consequences which affect the sitting balance, and also lead to reduced thoracic volume, reduced trunk height and development of pressure sores.

**Use of orthotics and its effect**: The type of orthotics used in children with myelomeningocele depends on the spinal level of lesion (Table 2). Their use in treatment regime is two-fold, one is to maintain posture or position due to paralysis of antigravity muscles and the second reason is to maintain correction after surgical procedures, most commonly after foot surgery.

Table 2.   Common orthotics used for different levels of defect.

| Level of MMCL | Type of Orthotic Used |
| --- | --- |
| 1. Lower Thoracic | Reciprocating gait orthotic (RGO) |
| 2. L1–L2 | Hip–Knee–Ankle–Foot orthotic (HKAFO) |
| 3. L3–L4 | Knee–Ankle–Foot orthotic (KAFO) |
| 4. L4–L5 | Foot orthotics or may not require orthotics |

## Fractures

Usually a fracture occurs below the neurological level and involves bone loss due to immobility. The most important aspect from the clinical point of view is that fractures in these children may not always present with pain. Signs of redness, warmth and occasional presence of crepitus should alert the treating physician of the possibility of fracture.

Knee and ankle fractures are most common and occur after development of contractures. Usually there is an exuberant growth of callus after fracture in bones complicated by neurological deficits and thus after healing the affected limb is bigger.

## Urological

### Introduction

It is fair to say that every child with a myelomeningocele will have a neurogenic bladder and not surprisingly, MMCL is the most common cause of neurogenic bladder in pediatric age group. Appropriate urological intervention is important in children with MMCL as urological dysfunction is a major long-term issue in these children from both medical and social points of view.

Normal bladder function depends on the interaction between

1. supraspinal structures: a paracentral lobe, second frontal gyrus and the Barrington center in the pontine reticular formation;
2. intraspinal structures: a sacral parasympathetic motor center (S2, S3, S4) and thoracolumbar sympathetic sensory center (T11, T12, L1 and L2).

Those two control centers are connected by vestibulospinal and corticospinal tracts.

Although it is intuitive to presume that only the spinal centers are affected in patients with spina bifida, it is currently believed that neurogenic bladder in MMCL is caused by upper and lower motor neuron lesion.

In this section we discuss the various urological aspects observed in spinal dysraphism, mainly focusing on myelomeningocele which constitutes almost 90% of all spinal dysraphism.

*Demography of urological complaints in myelomeningocele*

- All children born with myelomeningocele are considered to have neurogenic bladder with only 5% of children having normal voiding pattern by toilet-training age.

*Importance of early urological intervention*

The aim of early urological intervention is two-fold:

1. Prevent upper urinary tract (UUT) damage and resultant development of kidney dysfunction leading to ominous sign of chronic renal failure. This is the most important goal of treatment.
2. Improve the social aspect of life of children with MMCL by achieving sufficient bladder continence.

*Timing of visit to a urologist*

Urological management starts right after neurosurgical repair of myelomeningocele has been done. The manifestations of urological features vary considerably and cannot be predicted by either bony level of defect or by neurological examination.

However, the phenomenon of spinal shock occurring after the repair should be kept in mind before interpretation of any urological investigations. This clinical entity of spinal shock is transient and recovers usually within two to three weeks. Thus urological management starts right after repair of defect is undertaken.

*Radiological imaging*

- Incidence of hydronephrosis in infants is 7–31%
- Incidence of vesicoureteral reflux (VUR) is 20%

In the following image we observe:

1. A small, trabeculated bladder with multiple pseudodiverticula
2. Hydronephrosis seen on the left side with mildly tortuous and dilated ureter with blunting of pelvicalyceal system indicating grade 3 or 4 VUR.

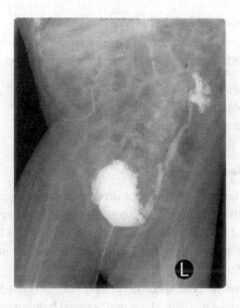

## Urodynamic findings

- Incidence of detrusor hypertonia/hypercontractility is 40–76%
- Incidence of areflexic bladder is about 26%

## Urological management

As a continuation of above discussion, urological management is instituted immediately after neurosurgical repair and will be discussed under the following headings:

i. Post-repair urological management
ii. Early urological management

i. *Post-repair urological management*

Immediately following repair of the defect, there is spinal shock with secondary flaccid bladder and urinary retention. Thus the treatment approach is intermittent catheterization till spontaneous voiding resumes. Most children resume normal spontaneous voiding pattern and then the following investigations are performed to form a baseline of urological function.

ii. *Early urological management*
   After the child recovers his or her normal voiding pattern, the following
   three baseline urological investigations are undertaken:

   • Urodynamic studies
   • Renal and bladder ultrasound
   • Voiding cystourethrogram (VCUG)

*Urodynamic studies*

From various studies it is evident that urodynamic testing can detect early
signs of cord dysfunction from subsequent tethering of spinal cord even
before radiological imaging or clinical examination. This clearly indicates
the importance of performing serial urodynamic studies in children with
myelomeningocele.

   The procedure is described here in brief. A catheter is inserted
transurethrally into the bladder, along with a rectal balloon for measurement
of intra-abdominal pressure. Contrast medium or saline is infused into the
bladder at a filling rate of 10% bladder capacity, simulating physiological
filling of bladder with urine. At the same time either patches of electrodes
or needle electrodes are placed in the perineum to measure external urethral
sphincter activity. Fluoroscopy is used to image the bladder outlet and detect
any reflux if present.

   In infancy, 12–32% of children are found to have normal urodynamic
condition. In 40–76% of children, detrusor hypercontractility is seen with
the rest having areflexic bladder.

   On the electromyography (EMG) studies of the external sphincter, 40%
have normal activity with 60% showing evidence of partial or complete denervation and another 10–54% showing incoordinate contraction between
the bladder and the sphincter, called *detrusor sphincter dysnergia.*

   Caution is advised while interpreting data from first urodynamic
evaluation as there can be artifacts from either the child being irritable or
immaturity of the nervous system. Thus the test should be repeated when
the child is calm.

   However, the following urodynamic parameter is used to classify
children into two categories and manage them accordingly. The leak point
pressure is considered a useful predictor of bladder dysfunction.

i. *High risk cases*

High risk infants are defined by the presence of detrusor sphincter dysnergia or presence of detrusor leak point pressure (OLPP, which is a measure of high intravesical pressure) more than 40 cm of $H_2O$.

Treatment: Start the child on anticholinergic medicine like oxybutynin to augment bladder emptying and also teach the parents on how to perform intermittent catheterization, every three hours during the day and once at least in the night time.

Vesicostomy is done only when there is intolerance or failure to treat by anticholinergics and there is persistence of increased detrusor pressure.

ii. *Low risk cases*

Low risk cases are defined as children with low DLPP, indicating near complete bladder emptying with resultant less intravesical pressure.

Treatment: Continue diaper drainage without intermittent catheterization up to six months of age. At this time perform urodynamic studies, along with VCUG and renal ultrasound to decide the treatment accordingly.

For low and high risk cases, perform urodynamic study, VCUG and renal ultrasound every six to eight months. Some prefer to perform urodynamic study annually and frequently only if new onset hydronephrosis, reflux UTI or febrile UTI develop.

*Role of antibiotic prophylaxis*

Children with any of the upper urinary tract changes like vesicoureteral reflux or development of hydronephrosis should be placed on antibiotics prophylaxis. However, the treating physician should always keep in mind that *asymptomatic bacteria*, which is defined as presence of cell count more than 100,000 in urine without any other signs of infection, is seen in 60–80% of children with myelomeningocele and neurogenic bladder. Antibiotic treatment is not needed in this case.

*Note on natural history of urological dysfunction in children with MMCL*

Maximum deterioration of urological function occurs within the first six months of age with the greatest concern being the denervation of the external sphincter, which will lead to fixed bladder outlet obstruction with subsequent deterioration of upper urinary tract.

Another study indicated that 32% of children who had low risk of UUT damage, i.e. low DLPP and normal UUT, progressed to high risk features such as high DLPP and abnormal UUT, within six months.

### *Explaining the deleterious effects of BOO (Bladder Outlet Obstruction)*

The pathophysiological aspects of bladder outlet obstruction and its consequences on evolution of irreversible kidney damage is described here.

The starting point of the cascade leading to renal damage is high intravesical pressure which impairs drainage of urine, leading to back pressure. The following are a brief account of this pathological process.

1. Intravesical pressure might arise from either hypertonic bladder contractions as a result of denervation or from detrusor sphincter dysnergia, which is explained as failure of receptive relaxation of the bladder neck and external urethral sphincter during the process of micturition, subsequently resulting in a functional bladder outlet obstruction.
2. Persistent high intravesical pressure, defined as pressure more than 40 cm of $H_2O$, can lead to increased voiding pressures (the bladder contracts forcefully, trying to overcome an abnormally closed sphincter to void urine).
3. The effect of this high intravesical pressure is decompensation of detrusor function which can be either areflexia from myogenic failure or resultant detrusor hypertrophy with formation of bladder sacculations and ultimately diverticula or trabulations. Either way, there is ineffective voiding ability of bladder and the result is increase in volume of residual urine.
4. The presence of residual urine becomes a nidus for infection which further compromises bladder function with inflammatory fibrotic process.
5. At this stage there is some element of mechanical ureterovesical junction obstruction which manifests as increased back pressure of urine and subsequent development of hydronephrosis.
6. With recurrent lower urinary tract infection and the development of significant vesicoureteral reflux (VUR), this becomes a convenient means of infected urine to reach the upper urinary tracts and the final

result is evolution of pyelonephritis and renal scarring, i.e. progression to renal failure.

## Mitrofanoff

It is a procedure that provides bladder augmentation with improvement in continence. A conduit, either appendix or ureter, is tunneled into the bladder in a non-refluxing flap valve technique. More than 90% of the patients achieve good continence with the Mitrofanoff procedure.

## Side effects

1. Stomal stenosis
2. Stones or bladder calculi
3. Foreign body reaction in the bladder
4. Hematoma and clot retention
5. May increase the risk of shunt infection through peritoneal catheter

## Causes of late deterioration of urological functions in a child with repaired myelomeningocele defect

Evidence of new onset or progression of denervation changes were detected in 50% of children and this was correlated with radiological evidence of tethering of the spinal cord. A subsequent untethering procedure led to improvement or stabilization of urological conditions in 90% of children.

Thus from the above discussion it is evident that tethering of spinal cord does have a deleterious effect on urological functions.

## Quality of life in children with spina bifida — coping with bowel and bladder issues

It has been observed that a bladder issue in children has a definite impact on the child's self-esteem and emotional outlook. However, it is important to differentiate conditions developing acutely versus onset of urinary complaints right from birth.

It has been noted that children with chronic illness scored higher than expected in many domains. One of the possible explanations given is that since the urinary issues have been present since birth, the child as well as the family have developed strategies to cope with this issue.

Children with higher maternal education and higher socioeconomic status (SES) faired better than foster kids. The explanation given is that children with higher SES had better motivation and resources to receive tertiary level care.

While assessing the impact of neurogenic bowel in children with myelomeningocele, there are two aspects which are taken into consideration:

1. *Severity of fecal incontinence*. It has two primary domains, which are the type and amount of stool loss.
2. *Quality of life and coping methods*. The common coping modalities include use of a pad or diaper.

The greater the degree of incontinence, the greater are the coping mechanism in the form of pads, diapers, enemas and other interventions leading to lifestyle changes.

Surprisingly, in some well-conducted studies it has been observed that there is a weak association between severity of fecal incontinence and health related quality of life (HRQOL) scores.

## Epilepsy

### Introduction

Seizures are not uncommon in children with myelomeningocele and especially when associated with hydrocephalus.

### Incidence

The following are series with reported incidence of seizures/epilepsy in children with myelomeningocele. The incidence ranges from 14.7–29% with MMCL and hydrocephalus as against 0–8% in children with MMCL and without hydrocephalus.

- From the abovementioned data, it is evident that hydrocephalus and shunt associated condition is an important and independent risk factor for seizures in children with myelomeningocele.
- Causes of seizures in myelomeningocele children with shunts:

  1. Minor cortical injury at the time of shunt insertion
  2. Shunt related issues like infection/malfunction

*Possible association of shunt and seizures*

1. Number of revisions — as the number of revisions increase so does the incidence of seizures from 5.9–24%
2. Infections like *Staphylococcus epidermidis*. In series by Blaauws, infection was associated with late onset epilepsy, with increase in incidence from 20% in non-infected shunts to 46% in infected shunts cases
3. There is a very weak correlation between ventricular catheter entry point and frequency of seizures, with only one study mentioned in the literature stating increased incidence of seizures with frontal entry point (54.5%) versus parietal entry point (6.6%)
4. No correlation between age at shunt insertion and seizure risk
5. Associated cerebral malformations

*Supratentorial anomalies in myelomeningocele as the etiology for seizures*

The presence of seizures in children with myelomeningocele before shunt insertion raises the question of cortical malformation as the main etiology for seizures.

The following are the types of cortical abnormalities implicated as causes of seizures in children with myelomeningocele with or without shunt, as shown by EEG studies.

1. **Polymicrogyria** (most common): a malformation where there is defect in neuronal migration resulting in small microgyri separated by shallow sulci and a slightly thickened cortex.
2. **Stenogyria**: presence of small, closely spaced gyri with no architectural abnormality; [Walpert *et al.*].
3. **Gray matter heterotopias**: failure of normal migration of neuroblast from the periventricular zone towards the cortex using the radial glia as their guide, resulting in abnormal cortical development and foci for epilepsy.

The most common type of crisis are generalized tonic-clonic and complex partial seizures. Usually monotherapy controls the seizures. It has been reported that 75% of patients with myelomeningocele and seizures were well-controlled with antiepileptic medicine.

It has to be reminded that development of seizures or non-response to therapy can herald a shunt malfunction. Often it is advised to revise the shunt even before presentation of classical symptoms of intracranial pressure.

## Obesity

Obesity in these children can lead to impairment of quality of life. The etiology of obesity is multifactorial and in this section we discuss the various morbidities associated with it.

### *Possible causes of obesity in children with myelomeningocele*

As mentioned above, the etiology of obesity is multifactorial with the following possible causes:

1. Endocrine malfunction
2. Metabolic syndrome
3. Decreased energy expenditure from immobility

### *Complications of obesity*

1. Limits use of wheelchair and orthoses
2. Difficult ambulation
3. Worsening of bowel and bladder incontinence
4. Worsening of decubitus ulcer

## Hematology

Deep vein thrombosis (DVT) is a common phenomenon seen in these children and is discussed here.

There are three important factors which increase the risk for DVT and they are all present in children with myelomeningocele. The factors are:

1. Immobility of lower limbs
2. Long hours of surgical procedure especially involving orthopedic and urological procedures
3. Obesity

## Sexual functions in men with MMCL

*Incidence of erectile dysfunction in men with MMCL*

About 40% of men with spina bifida engage in sexual activity at a mean age of 29 years. However, as high as 75% of these men have some form of erectile dysfunction. Erectile dysfunction is more commonly seen if the sacral reflexes are impaired. It has been noted that with level of T10 or lower, erection is possible but the primary dysfunction lies in maintaining erection. A short review of the male sexual function is described here.

*Physiology of penile erection*

Psychological, hormonal, vascular and neurological factors are involved in penile erection. The essential event is the vascular engorgement of the penis mediated by the pudendal arteries, which is in turn regulated by the thoracolumbar sympathetic outflow (T10–L2) and the sacral parasympathetic outflow (S2–S4).

Parasympathetic system responds to local tactile and psychological stimuli but the sympathetic system can only respond to psychological stimuli alone.

Penile erection is related to both sympathetic and parasympathetic nervous systems and intact tactile sensations indicate intact pudendal nerve function. However, the act of ejaculation is under the control of hypogastric nerve.

*Penile erection in men with MMCL*

Men with lesion T12 and below retain their psychogenic erectile ability even though the reflexogenic erectile ability is abolished. In this group of MMCL men, during the erection process, elongation and engorgement of penis is noted without sufficient rigidity. As these men have decreased or no intact tactile sensation of their penis, the primary erectile dysfunction in them is in the form of difficulty in maintaining erection.

The cerebral impulses travel down the thoracolumbar sympathetic outflow to the penis and mediate erection by inhibiting release of noradrenaline and increasing release of nitrous oxide and acetylcholine. As a result of decreased impulses traveling to the penis due to the absence of augmentation of the sacral impulses, erection is not strong enough.

*Management of erectile dysfunction in men with MMCL*

- Inhibit the action of phosphodiesterase and subsequently increase the release of nitrous oxide. The use of sildenafil (Viagra) which is a 5-phosphodiesterase inhibitor is advocated in men with MMCL.
- Always advise the patient to evacuate bowel and bladder before engaging in sexual intercourse.

## Suggested Readings

ACOG Practice Bulletin. Clinical management guidelines for obstetrician-gynaecologists. Replaces Committee Opinion Number 252, March 2001. Number 44, July 2003. *Obstet Gynaecol* 2003; **102**:203.

Adelberg A, Blotzer A, Koch G, Moise R, Chescheir N, Moise KJ Jr, Wolfe H. Impact of maternal-fetal surgery for myelomeningocele on the progression of ventriculomegaly *in utero. Am J Obstet Gynaecol* 2005 Sep; **193**(3 Pt 1):727–731.

Adzick NS, Sutton LN, Crombleholme TM, Flake AW. Successful fetal surgery for spina bifida. *Lancet* 1998; **352**:1675.

Barf HA, Verhoef M, Jennekens-Schinkel A, Post MW, Gooskens RH, Prevo AJ. Cognitive status of young adults with spina bifida. *Dev Med Child Neurol* 2003; **45**(12):813–820.

Bensen JT, Dillard RG, Burton BK. Open spina bifida: Does Cesarean section delivery improve prognosis? *Obstet Gynaecol* 1988 Apr; **71**(4):532–534.

Bowman RM, McLone DG, Grant JA, Tomita T, Ito JA. Spina bifida outcome: A 25-year prospective. *Pediatr Neurosurg* 2001; **34**(3):114–120.

Bowman RM, McLone DG. Tethered cord in children with spina bifida. *Spina bifida: Management and outcome*, Ozek MM (Ed), Springer, Milan 2008.

Bruner JP, Tulipan N, Paschall RL, Boehm FH, Walsh WF, Silva SR, Hernanz-Schulman M, Lowe LH, Reed GW. Fetal surgery for myelomeningocele and the incidence of shunt-dependent hydrocephalus. *JAMA* 1999 Nov 17; **282**(19):1819–1825.

Bruner JP. Intrauterine surgery in myelomeningocele. *Semin Fetal Neonatal Med* 2007 Dec; **12**(6):471–476.

Caines E, Dahl M, Holmström G. Long-term oculomotor and visual function in spina bifida cystic: Population-based study. *Acta Ophthalmol Scand* 2007; **85**:662–666.

Cass AS, Bloom BA, Luxenberg M. Sexual function in adults with myelomeningocele. *J Urol* 1986; **136**(2):425–426.

Chervenak FA, Duncan C, Ment LR, Tortora M, McClure M, Hobbins JC. Perinatal management of meningomyelocele. *Obstet Gynaecol* 1984; **63**(3):376–380.

Cohen AR, Robinson S. Early management of myelomeningocele. *Pediatric neurosurgery*, McLone DG (Ed), Saunders WB, Philadelphia 2001, p. 241.

Cremer R, Kleine-Diepenbruck U, Hoppe A, Blaker F. Latex allergy in spina bifida patients — prevention by primary prophylaxis. *Allergy* 1998; **53**(7):709–711.

Davis BE, Daley CM, Shurtleff DB, Duguay S, Seidel K, Loeser JD, Ellenbogan RG. Long-term survival of individuals with myelomeningocele. *Pediatr Neurosurg* 2005; **41**(4):186–191.

de Jong TH. Deliberate termination of life of newborns with spina bifida, a critical reappraisal. *Childs Nerv Syst* 2008; **24**(1):13–28.

Deprest JA, Done E, Van Mieghem T, Gucciardo L. Fetal surgery for anesthesiologists. *Curr Opin Anaesthesiol* 2008; **21**(3):298–307.

Dias MS. Neurosurgical causes of scoliosis in patients with myelomeningocele: An evidence-based literature review. *J Neurosurg* 2005; **103**:24–35.

Dik P, Klijn AJ, van Gool JD, de Jong-de Vos van Steenwijk CC, de Jong TP. Early start to therapy preserves kidney function in spina bifida patients. *Eur Urol* 2006; **49**(5): 908–913.

Doherty D, Shurtleff DB. Pediatric perspective on prenatal counseling for myelomeningocele. *Birth Defects Res A Clin Mol Teratol* 2006; **76**(9):645–653.

Dominic N, Thompson P. Postnatal management and outcome for neural tube defects including spina bifida and encephalocoeles. *Prenat Diagn* 2009 Feb 4.

Fletcher JM, Brookshire BL, Landry SH. Attentional skills and executive functions in children with early hydrocephalus. *Dev Neuropsychol* 1996; **12**:53.

Fichter MA, Dornseifer U, Henke J, Schneider KT, Kovacs L, Biemer E, Bruner J, Adzick NS, Harrison MR, Papadopoulos NA. Fetal spina bifida repair — current trends and prospects of intrauterine neurosurgery. *Fetal Diagn Ther* 2008; **23**(4):271–286.

Gardner P, Albright AL. Hereditary anterior sacral meningocele. *J Neurosurg* 2006; **104**(2):138–142.

Georgea TM, Cummings TJ. The immunohistochemical profile of the myelomeningocele placode: Is the placode normal? *Pediatr Neurosurg* 2003; **39**:234–239.

Harmon JP, Hiett AK, Palmer CG, Golichowski AM. Prenatal ultrasound detection of isolated neural tube defects: Is cytogenetic evaluation warranted? *Obstet Gynaecol* 1995; **86**(4 Pt 1):595–599.

Hopps CV, Kropp KA. Preservation of renal function in children with myelomeningocele managed with basic newborn evaluation and close followup. *J Urol* 2003; **169**(1):305–308.

Hill AE, Beattie F. Does Cesarean section delivery improve neurological outcome in open spina bifida? *Eur J Pediatr Surg* 1994; **4 Suppl 1**:32–34.

Holmbeck GN, Westhoven VC, Phillips WS, Bowers R, Gruse C, Nikolopoulos T, Totura CM, Davison K. A multimethod, multi-informant, and multidimensional perspective on psychosocial adjustment in preadolescents with spina bifida. *J Consult Clin Psychol* 2003; **71**(4):782–796.

Kessler TM, Lackner J, Kiss G, Rehder P, Madersbacher H. Predictive value of initial urodynamic pattern on urinary continence in patients with myelomeningocele. *Neurourol Urodyn* 2006; **25**(4):361–367.

Lewis D, Tolosa JE, Kaufmann M, Goodman M, Farrell C, Berghella V. Elective Cesarean delivery and long-term motor function or ambulation status in infants with meningomyelocele. *Obstet Gynaecol* 2004; **103**(3):469–473.

Lorber J. Spina bifida cystica. Results of treatment of 270 consecutive cases with criteria for selection for the future. *Arch Dis Child* 1972 Dec; **47**(256):854–873.

Marshall DF, Boston VE. Does the absence of anal reflexes guarantee a "safe bladder" in children with spina bifida? *Eur J Pediatr Surg* 2001; **11**(Suppl 1): S21–S23.

Matson MA, Mahone EM, Zabel TA. Serial neuropsychological assessment and evidence of shunt malfunction in spina bifida: A longitudinal case study. *Child Neuropsychology*, 2005; **11**:315–332.

McDonald CM, Jaffe KM, Mosca VS, Shurtleff DB. Ambulatory outcome of children with myelomeningocele: Effect of lower extremity muscle strength. *Dev Med Child Neurol* 1991; **33**(6):482–490.

Nelson MD, Widman LM, Abresch RT, Stanhope K, Havel PJ, Styne DM, McDonald CM. Metabolic syndrome in adolescents with spinal cord dysfunction. *J Spinal Cord Med* 2007; **30**:S127–S139.

Oakeshott P, Hunt GM, Whitaker RH, Kerry S. Perineal sensation: An important predictor of long-term outcome in open spina bifida. *Arch Dis Child*. 2007; **92**(1):67–70. Epub 2006 Aug 30.

Rintoul NE, Sutton LN, Hubbard AM. A new look at myelomeningoceles: Functional level, vertebral level, shunting, and the implications for fetal intervention. Pediatrics 2002; **109**(3):409–413.

Rendeli C, Nucera E, Ausili E, Tabacco F, Roncallo C, Pollastrini E, Scorzoni M, Schiavino D, Caldarelli M, Pietrini D, Patriarca G. Latex sensitization and allergy in children with myelomeningocele. *Childs Nerv Syst* 2006; **22**(1):28–32. Epub 2005 Feb 10.

Sakala EP, Andree I. Optimal route of delivery for meningomyelocele. *Obstet Gynaecol Surv* 1990; **45**(4):209–212.

Salomão F, Cavalheiro S, Matsushita H, Leibinger R, Bellas A, Vanazzi E, de Souza L, Nardi A. Cystic spinal dysraphism of the cervical and upper thoracic region; *Childs Nerv Syst* 2006; **22**:234–242.

Seitzberg A, Lind M, Biering-Sorensen F. Ambulation in adults with myelomeningocele. Is it possible to predict the level of ambulation in early life? *Childs Nerv Syst* 2008; **24**(2):231–237.

Shaer CM, Chescheir N, Schulkin J. Myelomeningocele: A review of the epidemiology, genetics, risk factors for conception, prenatal diagnosis, and prognosis for affected individuals. *Obstet Gynaecol Surv* 2007; **62**(7):471–479.

Singhal B, Mathew KM. Factors affecting mortality and morbidity in adult spina bifida. *Eur J Pediatr Surg* 1999; **9**(1):31–32.

Sival DA, Verbeek RJ, Brouwer OF, Sollie KM, Bos AF, den Dunnen WF. Spinal hemorrhages are associated with early neonatal motor function loss in human spina bifida aperta. *Early Hum Dev* 2008; **84**(7):423–431.

Stevenson KL. Chiari Type II malformation: Past, present, and future. *Neurosurg Focus* 2004 Feb 15; **16**(2):E5.

Sutton LN, Adzick NS, Bilaniuk LT, Johnson MP, Crombleholme TM, Flake AW. Improvement in hind-brain herniation demonstrated by serial fetal magnetic resonance imaging following fetal surgery for myelomeningocele. *JAMA* 1999 Nov 17; **282**(19):1826–1831.

Sutton LN. Fetal surgery for neural tube defects. *Best Pract Res Clin Obstet Gynaecol* 2008; **22**(1):175–188.

Swana HS, Sutherland RS, Baskin L. Prenatal intervention for urinary obstruction and myelomeningocele. *Int Braz J Urol* 2004; **30**(1):40–48.

Swank M, Dias LS. Walking ability in spina bifida patients: A model for predicting future ambulatory status based on sitting balance and motor level. *J Pediatr Orthop* 1994; **14**(6):715–718.

Tarcan T, Bauer S, Olmedo E, Khoshbin S, Kelly M, Darbey M. Long-term followup of newborns with myelodysplasia and normal urodynamic findings: Is followup necessary? *J Urol* 2001; **165**(2):564–567.

Trollmann R, Bakker B, Lundberg M, Doerr DH. Growth in pre-pubertal children with myelomeningocele (MMC) on growth hormone (GH): The KIGS experience. *Pediatric Rehabilitation* 2006; **9**(2):144–148.

Tubbs RS, Chambers MR, Smyth MD, Bartolucci AA, Bruner JP, Tulipan N, Oakes WJ. Late gestational intrauterine myelomeningocele repair does not improve lower extremity function. *Pediatr Neurosurg* 2003; **38**(3):128–132.

Tulipan N. Intrauterine myelomeningocele repair. *Clin Perinatol* 2003; **30**(3):521–530.

Tulipan N, Sutton LN, Bruner JP, Cohen BM, Johnson M, Adzick NS. The effect of intrauterine myelomeningocele repair on the incidence of shunt-dependent hydrocephalus. *Pediatr Neurosurg* 2003; **38**(1):27–33.

Verhoef M, Barf HA, Vroege JA. Sex education, relationships, and sexuality in young adults with spina bifida. *Arch Phys Med Rehabil* 2005; **86**(5):979–987.

Waters KA, Forbes P, Morielli A, Hum C, O'Gorman AM, Vernet O, Davis GM, Tewfik TL, Ducharme FM, Brouillette RT. Sleep-disordered breathing in children with myelomeningocele. *J Pediatr* 1998; **132**(4):672–681.

White DP. Pathogenesis of obstructive and central sleep apnea. *Am J Respir Crit Care* 2005; **172**:1363–1370.

Woodhouse CR. Myelomeningocele: Neglected aspects. *Pediatr Nephrol* 2008; **23**(8):1223–1231.

Yamada S, Won DJ, Yamada SM. Pathophysiology of tethered cord syndrome: Correlation with symptomatology. *Neurosurg Focus* 2004; **16**(2):E6.

Yoshida F, Morioka T, Hashiguchi K, Kawamura T, Miyagi Y, Nagata S, Mihara F, Ohshio M, Sasaki T, Epilepsy in patients with spina bifida in the lumbosacral region. *Neurosurg Rev* 2006; **29**:327–333.

Zolty P, Sanders MH, Pollack IF. Chiari malformation and sleep-disordered breathing: A review of diagnostic and management issues. *Sleep* 2000; **23**(5).

Chapter 5

# Occult Spinal Bifida

## Introduction

Occult spina bifida (SBO) represents failure of closure of the posterior neural arch, most commonly of the lumbar lamina with the underlying dura mater being intact and there is preservation of the underlying anatomy of the spinal cord. The possibility of this anomaly being present in completely asymptomatic individuals is high. In the great majority of cases the patient, or more correctly, the individual, is asymptomatic. But the term occult spina bifida has been subjected to a broader use of any spinal malformation which is covered with skin. This includes lesions other than myelomeningocele or lesion without the presence of exposed neural placode. The presence of skin markers in reality makes these lesions less occult in nature.

## Incidence

- Prevalence of SBO in the general population is:
  23% in England
  16.3% in Turkey
  18–34% in the United States
- SBO most frequently occurs in the lumbosacral spine, such as at L5, S1 or S2 alone or at S1 and S2.
- The condition is twice as common in males as in females.

Nonetheless, concerned clinicians have raised the question of whether spina bifida in children with lower urinary tract infection could be related to functional, not anatomical, anomaly of the spinal cord. While one group of investigators have concluded that constipation in children is associated with increased incidence of spina bifida occulta, the other group (Nejat F *et al.*), analyzing a larger number of patients, reached the following conclusions, "Among children with functional bowel and urinary problems, there was no statistically significant difference in the prevalence of abnormal spinal MR imaging findings in those with radiographic SBO and an age- and sex-matched control group. Spina bifida occulta was not shown to be a reliable indicator of spinal cord structural abnormalities. Its probable role as a finding associated with spinal cord dysfunction remains unclear."

But spina bifida occulta is also used in reference to all the cases that are not myelomeningocele, cases in which the patient's skin is intact over the observable defect. This is a misnomer that has persisted in medical terminology. Any of the following images are anything but occult. They all manifest to the trained eye that there has been a defect in the closure of the neural tube and that cutaneous ectoderm and neural ectoderm were not perfectly separated during the first month of intrauterine life.

## Skin Markers of Occult Spinal Dysraphism

Incidence of cutaneous lesions depicting an underlying occult spinal dysraphism ranges from 43–95%. A combination of two or more cutaneous signs is the strongest indicator of underlying occult spinal dysraphism. The following are the types of cutaneous markers for occult spinal dysraphism:

- Subcutaneous lipoma
- Dermal sinus
- Tail
- Dimple
- Localized hypertrichosis
- Hyperpigmented lesion

For these abovementioned skin lesions, a radiological imaging is always warranted. The specific lesions will be discussed in the corresponding sections.

## Mass at lumbosacral region

Presence of non-pulsatile, non-tender, soft lump at the lumbosacral area should raise the suspicion of an underlying spinal lipoma or lipomyelomeningocele.

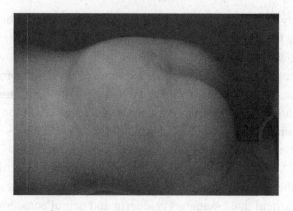

Isolated lipoma or lipoma occurring with other skin lesions like port wine stain (PWS) is the most common midline lesion associated with OSD. Presence of deviation of the gluteal cleft is another diagnostic marker indicative of an underlying mass, most commonly a lipomatous mass.

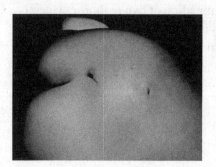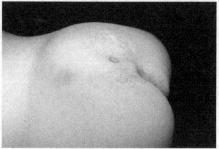

### Simple dimple vs. atypical dimple

Simple dimple is defined as a coccygeal pit of less than 5 mm in diameter and is located close to the anus, i.e. within 2.5 cm of the gluteal furrow or cleft. An isolated presence of simple dimple does not need further investigations. However presence of an atypical dimple which is characterized by size of more than 5 mm, located further than 2.5 cm from the anus and is also associated with other skin markers of OSD, definitely needs further investigations.

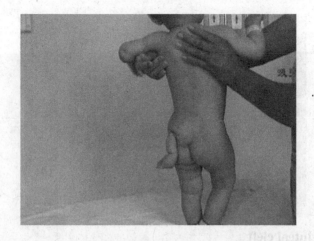

A tail or an appendix raises the question of NTD. A skin tag in the form of a human tail, known as neuroectodermal appendage, or a faun tail which is a tuft of coarse hair, surely does indicate underlying NTD.

## Hypertrichosis

This is almost a sure sign of diastematomyelia and has an incidence of 46–50%. It is most of the time in the form of a faun tail.

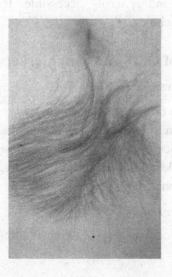

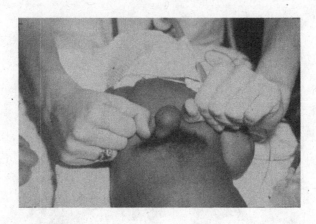

## Deviated gluteal cleft

This may be the only sign of underlying subcutaneous lipoma.

## Radiological Investigations

### Ultrasonography vs. MRI

Ultrasonography is the investigation of choice for infants of five to six months old, as the posterior elements of the infant spine ossifies by five to six months of age.

Advantages of ultrasound over MRI are — ultrasound is non-invasive, no sedation required and is easily accessible. However, MRI is the diagnostic modality of choice.

## Categories of Risk of OSD with Skin Markers

### High-risk skin markers

1. Combination of two or more skin lesions.
2. Presence of one skin lesion with signs of spinal cord dysfunction such as neurogenic bladder, or bowel and orthopedic signs.
3. Isolated cutaneous lesions which are highly suggestive of underlying OSD, including lipoma, dermal sinus or tail.

*Next step in management*

Undertake MRI examination of spine, even if ultrasound is negative of spinal dysraphism.

## Intermediate-risk skin markers

Presence of isolated skin markers like:

1. Aplasia cutis congenita
2. Deviated gluteal cleft
3. Atypical dimple

*Next step in management*

If the child is less than six months old, perform ultrasound and if it is positive then perform MRI. If the ultrasound is negative, no further examination is needed till six months of age when MRI can be undertaken then.

   If the child is older than six months, perform MRI examination.

## Low-risk skin markers

Presence of the following isolated skin lesions is rarely ever associated with occult spinal dysraphism:

1. Pigmented nevus
2. Simple dimple
3. Hemangioma
4. Mongolian spot

*Next step in management*

Usually no further investigation is required.

## Chapter 6

# Cervical Spinal Dysraphism

## Introduction

Unlike its lower lumbar counterpart, cervical spinal dysraphism has a surprisingly way better outcome in terms of neurological, orthopedic and urological issues. To begin with, the spinal dysraphism observed at the cervical level is more of a meningocele, defined as cystic protrusion of the meninges through the bony defect. However, the presence of some neural elements elude the use of the term *simple meningocele* but is known as *cervical MMCL*.

## Incidence

- Cervical spinal dysraphism accounts for 3.7% of neural tube defects.
- Mostly cervical spinal dysraphism is in the form of meningocele.
- About 5.5% of cases are occult with only cutaneous tell-tale signs of underlying spinal abnormality.
- Recurrence rate of 7.8% in siblings of cervical spinal dysraphism as compared to 0.7% recurrence rate in lower spina bifida.

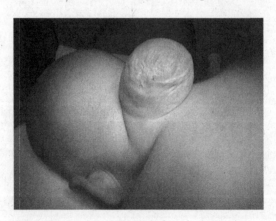

Concurrent lower spinal dysraphism is seen in a few cases which are mostly:

- Distematomyelia
- Tethered cord syndrome
- Lipomyelomeningocele
- Hydromyelia
- Thoracic hemivertebra

Associated upper spinal anomalies:

- Chiari malformation incidence of 44%
- Klippel–Feil deformity

## Clinical Features

The clinical feature varies from near normal neurological examination to deficits. These findings are described in the following section.

  i. Cutaneous findings
 ii. Infection
iii. Neurological findings

  i. *Cutaneous findings*
    Unlike their counterparts in the lumbosacral area, cervical dysraphism has a full-thickness skin covering the base with thick epithelium covering the surface.

    Other cutaneous signs indicative of underlying spinal pathology are as follows:

- Dimple
- Sinus
- Hairy patch
- Capillary nevus as seen in the following figure
- Congenital scar
- Lipoma

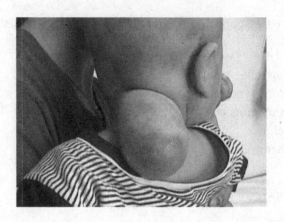

ii. *Infection*

  • Recurrent meningitis

iii. *Neurological findings*
    Symptoms in cervical dysraphism may range from minimal neurolog-
    ical impairment to cervical myelopathy. Presence of concurrent lower
    spinal defects further aggravates the clinical picture.
    *Symptoms*:

  • Upper limb paresis
  • Weakness and changes in deep tendon reflex in the lower limbs
    which is mostly asymmetrical
  • Gait abnormalities
  • Pyramidal signs like increased tone and brisk reflexes
  • Scoliosis
  • Sensory complaints of pain and paresthesias

## Outcome

  • Good prognosis of cervical dysraphism as compared to lower spinal
    defects with regards to neurological, orthopedic and urological systems.
  • Low incidence of hydrocephalus is seen.
  • About 40% improvements in clinical signs are seen in the postoperative
    period.
  • Intellectual and behavioral impairment is usually not seen.

## Thoracic dysraphism

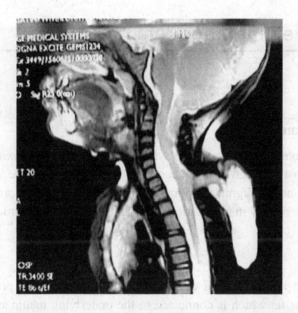

Also very rare, but in general good outcome. Notice in the figure the presence of descended cerebellar tonsils and medullary kinking, and a large sac with an exophytic stem of rudimentary nervous tissue.

## Chapter 7

# Lipomyelomeningocele

## Introduction

The term lipomyelomeningocele is synonymous with the term *spinal lipoma* and is the most common form of occult spinal dysraphism. In the absence of obvious cutaneous stigmata, lipomyelomeningocele can have a late onset of symptoms mainly in association with tethering of spinal cord.

## Definition

Lipomyelomeningocele is a condition characterized by the presence of subcutaneous fat which is connected to the underlying meninges and the open neural placode through a deficient lumbodorsal fascia and non-fused posterior vertebral arches. The anatomical defect is akin to myelomeningocele except that the lesion is skin-covered, which is indicative of the fact that the defect occurred after closure of neural tube (limited myeloschisis).

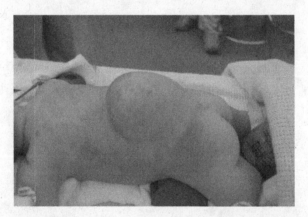

From the clinical point of view, the presence of fat in the cord leads to the phenomenon of tethered cord syndrome. Usually a lipomyelomeningocele tethers the cord asymmetrically with rotation of the cord and subsequently leads to asymmetrical length of nerve roots with the shorter roots on the side of the lipoma. This finding is also corroborated with more severe neurological deficits on the ipsilateral side of the lipoma.

## Incidence and Prevalence

The true incidence of this congenital anomaly cannot be assessed due to its occult nature, i.e. the patient can remain totally asymptomatic. Thus the advent of MRI imaging in 1986 has helped to detect and visualize this condition better.

Incidental findings in autopsy of adults are 5% while incidence in live births is approximately 1 in 4000. The ratio of female to male is 2:1, indicating that this condition is more common in females. The most common site of involvement is the lumbosacral region.

## Inheritance Pattern

Most cases of lipomyelomeningocele are sporadic in nature, with very few cases report of hereditary trait of presentation and they were all autosomal recessive form of inheritance. The next question is: Will future pregnancies be affected? The recurrent risk of lipomyelomeningocele is seen to be minimal with 4% risk in siblings of proband.

## Embryology

While comparing lipomyelomeningocele with its more severe counterpart, the myelomeningocele, it is more than evident that they differ not only in the clinical outcome but also from the embryo genetic point of view. A famous study from Nova Scotia, Canada, demonstrated the apparent failure of preconception folic acid in preventing or even declining the incidence of lipomyelomeningocele. This impelling evidence indicates the heterogeneity of the clinical manifestation of spinal dysraphism. Lipomyelomeningocele is hypothesized to arise during the period of canalization of the tail bud, i.e. day 28 to 48 of gestation. The origin of adipocytes or fat cells within the spinal column in association with closed spinal dysraphism has led to many theories of the pathogenesis of lipomyelomeningocele and some of them are described here briefly.

**Virchow, Chiari and Von Recklinghausen theory**

According to these physicians, they regarded the origin of lipomas in the spine to be normal adipocytes present in meninges during the postnatal life. However, this theory could not explain the consistent dorsal nature of the spinal lipomas and also failed to explain the universal lumbosacral location of the lipoma.

**Taubner theory**

According to Taubner, spinal lipomas represented fatty degeneration of glial cells present within the meninges and these degenerated cells could be identified by the accumulation of fats in their cytoplasm. However, from histopathological studies it was proven that the fats in these spinal lipomas are not consequences of fatty degeneration. On the other hand, the histology of spinal lipomas shows presence of mature adipose tissue and there was no evidence of fatty degeneration.

**Ehni and Love theory**

These two physicians proposed the cell of origin of adipocytes in spinal lipomas to be the primitive vascular mesoderm. They stated that the vascular mesoderm is capable of differentiating into adipose tissue but is inhibited from doing so under the influence of neural crest cells. Again the theory could not explain the typical location of the lipomas. Combined embryological and cytochemical studies revealed that mesodermal cells differentiate into vascular mesoderm and not adipocytes.

**McLone and Naidich theory**

It took nearly half a century to delineate the pathogenesis of this category of NTD and so far this has been the most widely accepted theory explaining lipomyelomeningocele. According to McLone and Naidich, the process of non-disjunction or premature separation of the neuroectodermal tissue from the surrounding cutaneous ectodermal tissue results in the neural plate being exposed posteriorly. This subsequently allows the paraxial mesoderm to invade the neural cleft with the exuberant growth of the heterotrophic fatty mesenchyme, which becomes an obstacle in the proper closure of the neural tube. In other words, this leads to a state of partial dorsal myeloschisis and the resultant occurrence of lipomyelomeningocele.

The internal or luminal surface of the ectoderm induces the mesenchyme to differentiate into adipose tissue and the external ectoderm covers the incompletely closed neural tube to form pia-arachnoid and dura mater. This hypothesis comes from the observation of histological section from spinal lipomas revealing a multitude of tissues arising from all three germ layers. The presence of epithelia of various types, mesodermal tissues such as striated muscle fibers, has been documented. This pathological analysis of the tissue further emphasizes the non-disjunction of the cutaneous ectoderm from the neural ectoderm with the growth of the intervening mesenchyme. The process seems to occur during the period from the onset of closure of the neural tube by primary neurulation to the completion of secondary neurulation.

## Classification (by Chapman)

### Dorsal lipomyelomeningocele

In this variant the subcutaneous lipoma penetrates the fascia and the posterior elements to attach to the dorsal aspect of the descended conus medullaris. Often there is presence of a thickened or fatty filum terminale. The conus, dura mater and the lipoma unite along the edge of the neural ridges with the sensory roots exiting just lateral to this union.

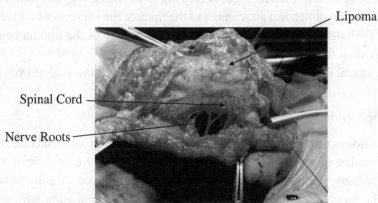

## Caudal lipomyelomeningocele

In this variant the lipoma attaches to the inferior aspect of the conus and extends to the central canal. There may be presence of nerve roots within the lipoma which might require surgical untethering.

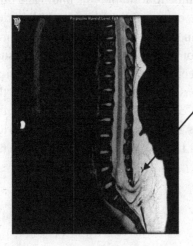

Lipoma with lumbar nerve roots spread into the fatty tissue

## Transitional lipoma

This variant of lipomyelomeningocele has features of both the above-mentioned types, i.e. dorsal and caudal variants with the lipoma extending into the central canal. Transitional lipoma has a large neural placode–lipoma interface with asymmetrical attachment, with more lipomas predominate on the left side and the meninges herniating to the right side. In cases with significant asymmetrical attachment of the lipoma, the nerve roots will also differ by length, with the roots on the ipsilateral side of the lipoma being shorter than the contralateral side. Henceforth, there is asymmetry of the neurological deficits with more pronounced deficits on the side of lipoma.

## Histopathology

Lipomatous component consists of mature adipocytes with metabolic rate same as that of adipocytes outside of the spinal cord or elsewhere in the body, which is adult yellow fat with occasional presence of baby brown fat. The fat content increases in proportion of fat accumulation with age.

Malignant transformation of the lipoma in the spine is almost never seen. From pathological studies of excised lipoma from surgical untethering procedures, tissues from different germ cell layers are found at times like muscle fibers, cartilage and neural tissue. This raises the question of whether the lumbosacral lipoma actually represents a form of teratoma. There are also cases that report spinal lipoma with concurrent presence of teratoma. This would involve a slightly different embryological origin of spinal lipomas, probably from some embryonic multipotent cell lineage. However, more evidence is needed to support this theory.

## Associated Pathological Features

### Spinal malformations

Other than the clinical manifestations of tethered cord syndrome, there are additional spinal pathologies that further aggravate the clinical picture:

1. Low lying conus medullaris
2. Malformed cauda equina
3. Syringomyelia
4. Diastematomyelia
5. Dural malformations

### 1. Low lying conus medullaris
The presence of a medullary conus below L2 of vertebral body is considered low lying conus. This radiological finding is seen in 72–94% of cases, making it undoubtedly the most common pathology. As we will see in the forthcoming sections, lipomyelomeningocele is also the most common condition leading to tethered cord syndrome.

### 2. Malformed cauda equina
Due to the presence of fatty tissue within the spinal cord, there is some anomalous development of the exiting caudal spinal nerve roots, especially with the rotated conus. The lipoma is thus unequally situated and the clinical consequence of this pathology is asymmetrical neurological deficits, more pronounced on the side of the lipoma.

### 3. Syringomyelia

Fluid filled cavitations within the spinal column is called *syringomyelia.*
This pathology is commonly associated with neural tube defects. The syrinx
is seen most commonly with transitional type of lipomyelomeningocele.
Such syringes are caudal in location and extend for only two to three spinal
levels. Patients with syringes tend to be symptomatic earlier and with more
progressive symptoms. The precise etiology is not well understood but it
seems to be more related to the tethered cord than to the presence of lipoma
mass in itself.

### 4. Diastematomyelia

Diastematomyelia or split cord malformation is a type of neural tube
defect involving the duplication of the spinal cord which are separated
from each other by presence of a median osseous or fibro-osseous septum.
This pathology may be concurrently seen in 9–27% of cases coexisting
with lipomyelomeningocele. The very fact of coexistence of multiple
pathologies in spinal dysraphism cases clearly indicates the importance and
the rational of evaluating children with spina bifida by MRI investigations
of the spine.

### 5. Dural malformations

With the anomalous development of the conus in spinal lipoma cases,
abnormalities arising in the meningial coverings like the dura mater are
commonly noted. The following are common dural pathologies seen:

  i. Dermal sinus tract
 ii. Teratoma
iii. Dural AVM
 iv. Dermoid or epidermoid cyst

i. *Dermal sinus tract*: An epithelium-lined tract extending from the skin
to deeper tissues is a dermal sinus tract. It arises from the defective
separation of the cutaneous ectoderm from the underlying neuroectoderm.
The implication of this benign developmental anomaly is the associated
infectious and neurological complications in the form of abscess and
tethering of spinal cord, respectively.

ii. *Teratoma*: Teratoma is a multilineage congenital tumor with presence
of tissues originating from all three germ cell layers.

iii. *Dural arteriovenous malformation* (*AVM*): This is a rare association seen with spinal lipomas but nevertheless has a highly morbid outcome from ruptures of the vascular malformation and concurrent damage to the cord.

iv. *Enteric dermoid or epidermoid*: Both dermoid and epidermoid cyst are congenital tumor and are at times associated with spinal lipomas.

## Vertebral anomalies

The bony anomalies arising from primary neurulation defect also affects the development of the adjacent somites which are the future vertebral bodies. These vertebral defects are delineated clearly in X-ray examination and are observed as bifid vertebrae (hemivertebrae), presence of vertebral body fusion and sacral aplasia or agenesis. These bony anomalies may also cause scoliosis in these patients. However, the primary cause of scoliosis in children with spina bifida is still syringomyelia.

## Visceral malformation

Common visceral malformations seen in children with spinal lipoma are mostly of anorectal and urological system involvement like imperforate anus. The reported incidence of these malformations range from 16–27%. The reason behind this association has been attributed to the anomalous development of caudal eminence and its derivatives.

## Brain anomalies

There is a very weak association between closed lower spinal dysraphism and brain anomalies with few case reports in the medical literature. They include Chiari malformation, hydrocephalus and presence of intracranial lipomas. The reason behind these associations is yet to be defined.

## Clinical Presentation

### Age of presentation

There is a bimodal age of presentation of spinal lipomas with the first peak in infancy followed by the second peak at the adolescent age group of 10 to 12 years. The reason behind this bimodal age distribution is explained as follows. In the infancy period it is usually a consultation with a pediatrician regarding the presence of a cutaneous marker on the skin of lower back when spinal lipomas are discovered. However, there are cases where the cutaneous markers are absent or are inconspicuous. Then during their adolescent age such children present most commonly with urological or neuro-orthopedic complaints. An MRI imaging of the spine is all that is needed to highlight the phenomenon of the underlying occult spinal dysraphism and the associated tethered cord syndrome.

### Clinical presentations of spinal lipomas

Usually children born with spinal lipoma are asymptomatic at birth and only the presence of various types of cutaneous markers indicate the underlying spinal dysraphism.

### Cutaneous markers

In as many as 90% of cases with spinal lipoma, there are cutaneous markers present that indicate the underlying pathology. More than half of the cases have multiple cutaneous markers.

- Midline or paraspinal mass
- Derivation of the gluteal furrow
- Changes in skin pigmentation (port wine stain) or skin tags
- Hirsutism/hypertrichosis (tufts of hair)
- Dimple
- Dermal sinus
- Rudimentary tail or an appendage
- Atretic meningocele
- Capillary hemangioma/telangiectasia

Out of the abovementioned types of cutaneous markers, it is the subcutaneous lipoma that is most commonly associated with spinal lipoma and is seen in almost 60% of cases. Some images have been introduced in the previous chapter. There is no typical image of a spinal lipoma.

## Examination of subcutaneous mass in infant with spinal lipoma

Mass is completely covered with full-thickness skin and is located usually in the midline but occasionally can be eccentric in position. Asymmetrical mass is usually seen in more than one-third of cases and the neurological deficits are more pronounced ipsilateral to the subcutaneous mass. The mass is non-tender. There is preservation of normal gluteal fold and when the gluteal fold is obscured or distorted then probability of concurrent occurence of myelocystocele should be taken into consideration. At times the presence of coccygeal pit overlying the coccyx with preservation of the intergluteal cleft is observed.

## Neurological Features

### Age of presentation

Children born with spinal lipoma are completely asymptomatic at birth with only cutaneous markers as evidence of the underlying spinal defect. In the past, with conservative treatment of these asymptomatic children with spinal lipomas, it was observed that a large percentage of children became symptomatic by 10–12 years of age. This also coincided with periods of rapid skeletal growth seen during onset of puberty. It was observed from patient records that transitional lipomas had worse outcomes than caudal and dorsal lipomas.

### Common precipitating factors

During full flexion movement of the neck there is a sudden upward movement of the spine by 2 cm. Thus any activity with prolonged flexion-extension movements of the spine such as gymnastics, ballet dancing and knee chest bends would lead to abrupt onset of clinical symptoms. These clinical symptoms include:

1. Pain
2. Sensorimotor complaints
3. Neuro-orthopedic complaints
4. Urological complaints

## 1. Pain

Children with spinal lipomas usually present with vague complaints of pain. Pain is usually felt at the lower back, with rarely ever at the perineal region which is common in adulthood presentation. The pain is often described as being dysesthetic in quality and ill-localized with occasional radiation to legs. The distribution of pain is non-dermatomal and is aggravated further by flexion-extension movements of spine.

A characteristic clinical feature which distinguishes pain of tethered cord syndrome from discogenic pain caused by damaged intervertebral disc is that the pain in tethered cord syndrome is not relieved by rest or supine position. In fact, in supine position the lumbar and cervical curvatures diminish and this leads to lengthening of the cord and increases the traction of the tethered cord.

## 2. Sensorimotor complaints

The sensorimotor findings are described according to age of presentation.

*Infants*: A detailed neurological examination in infants is not very conclusive as many of the positive findings are masked by the immaturity of the developing nervous system. However, the following are signs one should look out for while examining an infant with presence of a subcutaneous mass and possibility of underlying spinal dysraphism.

i. *Muscle bulk*: Decrease in the bulk of muscles or atrophy of muscles is masked in infants by the presence of baby fat or brown fat. However, one can look for obvious atrophy of muscle in the lower limbs by inspection of the calf, buttocks and the hollow of foot. Presence of atrophy is indicative of lower motor neuron dysfunction and injury to the alpha motor neuron in the ventral horns of the spinal gray matter.

ii. *Posture and tone*: In an infant one should look for posture and spontaneous movements of legs. Inspect the foot for presence of plantar creases. These creases indicate the functional integrity of plantar-flexors group of muscles which correlates with spinal level of S1 functionality.

iii. *Developmental milestones*: Examination for detecting gross motor skills like the ability to stand, crawl or walk should be conducted.

iv. *Examination of spine and foot*: Look for obvious deformities of spine and foot which would include asymmetrical length of lower limbs. Inspect foot for deformities like pes cavus, which is foreshortening of foot and is commonly seen in spinal lipoma.

*Older children*: Usually late onset of symptoms of spinal lipoma is manifested as neuro-orthopedic or urological complaints. In addition, these children lack the cutaneous markers associated with lipomyelomeningocele or even if present, they are very inconspicuous and thus escaped detection earlier. With increasing age there is a neurological picture of combined upper motor and lower motor neuron dysfunction. This combined picture is explained by the dysfunction of long tracts like the corticospinal tract, along with ventral horn dysfunction representing lower motor neuron dysfunction and is strongly associated with tethered cord syndrome.

The presence of the lipoma leads to local compression of the cord and mass effect as well as tethers or fixates the cord, thus preventing its natural physiological ascent with growth, subsequently leading to traction injury of the lumbosacral cord. In essence there is tethering of cord.

Clinically these lesions present with asymmetrical weakness and unequal length of legs.

i. *Motor examination*: Parents or teachers in school notice that the child is slower than his or her peers in sports or when running, jumping or hopping. Decreased tone presenting with flaccid weakness of legs always points towards dysfunction at lumbosacral segment. Subtle weaknesses in lower limbs become evident when the child is asked to hop or skip. Weakness while climbing down stairs is indicative of quadriceps weakness as the knee cannot lock and stiffen to gain stability. Spinal level considered is L2 to L5.

Weakness while climbing up stairs is indicative of weakness of hip extensors. Spinal level considered is L1 to L4. Inability to walk on toes is indicative of weakness of gastrocnemius-soleus muscle which is the main plantar flexors of the foot. The gastrocnemius-soleus muscles are innervated by S1. Inability to walk on heels is indicative of weakness of the anterior tibialis muscle, the main dorsiflexors of foot. The muscles of the anterior compartment of the leg including the anterior tibialis muscle are innervated by spinal level L5.

In lower motor neuron lesions, these deep tendon reflexes are decreased while in lesion of upper motor neuron the reflexes are brisk. Presence of clonus with increased spasticity of lower legs with secondary scissoring gait is highly indicative of corticospinal tract dysfunction secondary to spinal cord tethering. The selective susceptibility of corticospinal tracts to ischemia is explained by the fact that thick myelinated fibers like the corticospinal tracts require more vascular supply than thin unmyelinated fibers. This also represents a possible role of ischemia in tethered cost syndrome.

ii. *Gait*: Stumbling while walking is an early indicator of weakness of evertors and dorsiflexors of foot correlating with spinal level L5. Clinically such weakness manifests with dragging of the foot while walking. The child is often described as clumsy and falls frequently. After some time the parents note an increase in falling on even surfaces which are described as "tripping without any cause". An aftermath of this frequent falling is sprains and injuries indicative of gait instability.

### 3.  Neuro-orthopedic problems

With spinal lipomas or closed spinal dysraphism, the orthopedic complaints are much less severe as compared to its open counterpart, i.e. myelomeningocele. The new onset of neuro-orthopedic syndrome or deterioration of any pre-existing deficit should alert the treating physician of the possibility of tethered cord syndrome or re-tethering of previously operated spinal lipoma. Neuromuscular imbalance resulting in abnormal activation of agonist and antagonist muscles is responsible for orthopedic complaints seen in these cases.

*Foot deformity*

Progressive talipes or walking on toes is the most common lesion. The mildest form of talipes is hammer toes, i.e. fixed flexion at interphalangeal joint with extension at metatarsal phalangeal joint. Forefoot valgus, meaning out-turned foot, and varus deformity (in-turned foot), are frequently seen. Pes cavus, i.e. exaggerated horizontal or vertical pedal arches along with equino calcaneal varus deformity, also called club foot, is among other foot deformities seen. Club foot includes the following abnormalities: forefoot adduction, plantar flexion and internal rotation. Joint defects like subluxation of hip joint or asymmetrical length of legs are also seen.

*Scoliosis*

Progressive scoliosis with occasional presence of kyphosis is observed. Significant scoliosis is defined as when the curvature angle is more than

30° to 40°. However, before undertaking orthopedic correction of scoliosis, first, one has to rule out tethered cord.

## 4. Urological complaints
### *Bowel and bladder dysfunction*

Dysfunction of lower urinary tract, including the sphincters of both the bladder and bowel, has been noted in tethered cord syndrome due to spinal lipoma. The clinical manifestation is in the form of delayed toilet training or nocturnal enuresis. The other clinical features include:

- Urge and stress incontinence
- Urgency and frequency
- Poor voluntary control
- Post-void dribbling
- Frequent urinary tract infections

However, it has been noted that at times the only neurological abnormality may be evident from an abnormal urodynamic evaluation, as urological complaints are usually masked in infants and cannot be assessed by clinical examination alone. This clearly indicates the importance of performing urodynamic studies in all children presenting with suspected lipomyelomeningocele. Common urodynamic findings in children with spinal lipomas are discussed below.

i.    *Flaccid bladder*: Flaccid bladder with significant post-void volume arises when the parasympathetic center in the sacral segment called the Onuf's nucleus is affected, resulting in weakening of the detrusor muscle. Secondarily there is poor emptying of bladder and sensation of incomplete voiding.

ii.    *Detrusor sphincteric dysnergia*: Detrusor sphincter dysnergia or DSD is explained as areflexic but hypertonic bladder, arising due to dysfunctional descending corticospinal pathways and sacral segments. When there is abnormal simultaneous activation of the pudendal nucleus (external sphincter) and pelvic nucleus (detrusor) resulting in contracting bladder against a closed sphincter, the pathology is described as detrusor sphincter dysnergia and it is often complicated by a 50% chance of developing reflux and hydronephrosis. This is the most ominous sign of bladder dysfunction as it often leads to upper renal tract damage.

iii. *Uninhibited bladder contractions with hypertonic detrusor*: Sympathetic innervations are the first to be affected in tethered cord with subsequent development of non-functional internal sphincter with sagging of the proximal urethra and effacement of the bladder neck. The result is post-void dribbling and stress incontinence, which are early signs of neuropathic bladder.

## Natural History of Lipomyelomeningocele

The concept that children with lipomyelomeningocele are asymptomatic at birth is changing because it is difficult to elicit subtle neurological signs in children, as the signs are masked by neuronal plasticity.

The earliest signs that are seen are demonstrated by urodynamic studies and most of the time the signs are abnormal. Untreated cases can potentially lead to progressive neurological damage due to cord tethering, which subsequently leads to traction and ischemic injury of cord, especially during rapid growth phases such as puberty. Thus there is a general consensus that prophylactic surgery for these patients prevents damaged cord from tethering.

## Diagnostic Imaging

### Antenatal diagnosis

It is usually difficult to detect spinal lipoma antenatally especially in the presence of normal level of alpha feto protein in maternal serum.

*Ultrasonography*: By conducting prenatal ultrasound between 17th and 26th week of pregnancy, lipomyelomeningocele can be diagnosed based on the following features:

- Lumbosacral spina bifida
- Hypoechogenic area consistent with meningocele
- Overlying hyperechogenic skin
- No hydrocephalus

### Postnatal imaging

*X-ray*: Due to the presence of multiple ossification centers in neonates and infants, X-ray is not very conclusive and considered rather obsolete.

*CT myelogram*: This investigation helps to delineate the ventral surface of the spinal cord and the exiting nerve roots. But due to its invasive nature and with the advent of MRI, this test is no longer recommended.

*Spinal ultrasound*: Spinal ultrasound is the screening investigation of choice for detecting spinal lipomas up to six months of age as it is non-invasive. It should be performed on every neonate even for asymptomatic ones with cutaneous stigmata of occult spina bifida. Presence of homogeneous, well-demarcated, intraspinal hyperechogenic (more echogenic than epidural fat) mass with findings of spinal defects is a sure diagnosis of lipomyelomeningocele.

*MRI of lumbosacral spine*: MRI of spine without contrast is sufficient enough to clearly reveal the underlying pathology of the anomalous spinal development. Fat has a short relaxation time and thus appear with high signal intensity on T1 weighted MRI image. Visualization in both sagittal and axial planes of MRI will precisely reveal the lipoma and its association with adjacent structures. The diagnosis of tethered cord also involves location of the conus, i.e. whether it is low lying or not.

## Definitions of Variants of Spinal Dysraphism Associated with Spinal Lipoma

The following are two variants of closed neural tube defect associated with presence of fat or spinal lipoma.

### Lipomyelocele/Lipomyeloschisis

A lipoma which attaches to the open neural placode within the confines of the spinal canal is called *lipomyelocele* or the old term *lipomyeloschisis*. This condition is twice as common as the lipomyelomeningocele.

### Lipomyelocystocele

A lipoma which is associated with dilatation of the terminal portion of central canal into an ependymal lined cyst that does not communicate with the subarachnoid space is called *lipomyelocystocele*.

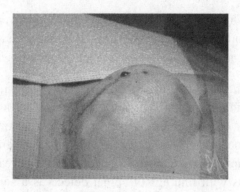

The appearance of the above lesion is similar to that of any other lipoma. In the image below the dome of the lipoma has already been exposed. Underneath it the terminal portion of the central canal can be seen.

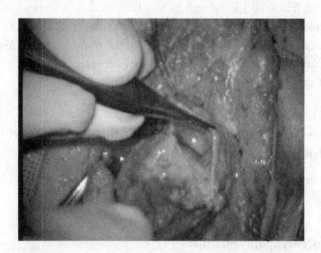

## Surgery

The two indications for surgery are to prevent tethering of the cord and to remove a stigmatizing lesion. It seems clear and simple but the truth is that the issue regarding surgical indications for lipomas is not settled.

We are all aware of patients with tethered cord who had a partial surgery for their lipomas. Usually they had a surgery limited to removing the subcutaneous fat and dividing the stem of the lipoma before it entered, or exited, the dura mater. The lipoma that was adhered to the cord was left intact. Those patients come to our clinic because they have symptoms related to tethering of the cord. On the other hand we do see our own patients who, in spite of having had surgery in which the intradural lipoma was partially removed, they do return with the same symptoms as those whose surgery was less ambitious.

Those patients whom we could not help raise questions on our own abilities, or on the correctness of the indication for surgery.

The group from Hopital Necker in Paris has stepped forward in this matter and has proposed that we should refrain from operating any asymptomatic patient with a lumbosacral lipoma, with the exception of those with thickened filum terminale. Dr Pierre Kahn and his group, all highly respected pediatric neurosurgeons, support their suggestion with evidence that surgery does more harm than good. These physicians put forth the argument that as the natural history of the disease is uncertain, we should not rush into surgery to operate on a child who does not have symptoms. This approach is also followed by other medical centers such as the Hospital Garrahan in Buenos Aires.

Although expectant treatment for spinal lipomas is a possible treatment option, I believe that each patient is unique, even when the individual seems to share radiological and clinical characteristics with a myriad of other patients. With adequate surgical technique, and with adequate intra-operative monitoring and with the understanding that sometimes the surgery will not reach half of its objectives, every patient with a lipoma should be given the chance to have the risk of tethered cord reduced, if not eliminated.

It is in matters like this that the two personalities of medicine, the Art and the Science, should have equal weight in the discussion. Thus we shall leave the final decision on surgical indication of each case to each particular surgeon. Lastly, let us not forget that medicine is a constantly evolving science that searches innovative treatments on the shoulders of its failures.

## Suggested Readings

Barolat G, Schaefer D, Zeme S. Recurrent spinal cord tethering by sacral nerve root following lipomyelomeningocele surgery. *J Neurosurg* 1991; **75**:143–145.

Blount JP, Elton S. Spinal lipomas. *Neurosurg Focus* 2001; **10**(1):Article 3.

Colak A, Pollack IF, Albright AL. Recurrent tethering: A common long-term problem after lipomyelomeningocele repair. *Pediatr Neurosurg* 1998; **29**:184–190.

Finn MA, Walker ML. Spinal lipomas: Clinical spectrum, embryology, and treatment. *Neurosurg Focus* 2007; **23**(2):E10.

Fone PD, Vapnek JM, Litwiller SE, *et al.* Urodynamic findings in the tethered spinal cord syndrome: Does surgical release improve bladder function? *J Urol* 1997; **157**: 604–609.

Foster LS, Kogan BA, Cogen PH, *et al.* Bladder function in patients with lipomyelomeningocele. *J Urol* 1990; **143**:984–986.

Gower DJ, Engles CF, Friedman ES. Thoracic intraspinal lipoma. *Br J Neurosurg* 1994; **8**:761–764.

Hoffman HJ, Taecholarn C, Hendrick EB, *et al.* Management of lipomyelomeningoceles. Experience at the Hospital for Sick Children, Toronto. *J Neurosurg* 1985; **62**:1–8.

Kanev PM, Bierbrauer KS. Reflections on the natural history of lipomyelomeningocele. *Pediatr Neurosurg* 1995; **22**:137–140.

Kannu P, Furneaux C, Aftimos S. Familial lipomyelomeningocele: A further report. *Am J Med Genet* 2005; **132A**:90–92.

La Marca F, Grant JA, Tomita T, *et al.* Spinal lipomas in children: Outcome of 270 procedures. *Pediatr Neurosurg* 1997; **26**:8–16.

McLone DG, Naidich TP. Laser resection of fifty spinal lipomas. *Neurosurgery* 1986; **18**:611–615.

McNeely PD, Howes WJ. Ineffectiveness of dietary folic acid supplementation on the incidence of lipomyelomeningocele: Pathogenetic implications. *J Neurosurg* 2004; **100**(2):98–100.

Peter JC. Occult dysraphism of the spine. A retrospective analysis of 88 operative cases, 1979–1989. *S Afr Med J* 1992; **81**:351–354.

Pierre-Kahn A, Lacombe J, Pichon J. Intraspinal lipomas with spina bifida. Prognosis and treatment in 73 cases. *J Neurosurg* 1986; **65**:756–761.

Pierre-Kahn A, Zerah M, Renier D, Cinalli G, Sainte-Rose C, Lellouch-Tubiana A, Brunelle F, Merrer ML, Giudicelli Y, Pichon J, Kleinknecht B, Nataf F. Congenital lumbosacral lipomas. *Child's Nerv Syst* 1997; **13**:298–335.

Rappaport ZH, Tadmor R, Brand N. Spinal intradural lipoma with intracranial extension. *Child's Brain* 1982; **9**:411–418.

Satar N, Bauer SB, Shefner J. The effects of delayed diagnosis and treatment in patients with an occult spinal dysraphism. *J Urol* 1995; **154**:754–758.

Souweidane MM, Drake JM. Re-tethering of sectioned fibrolipomatous filum terminales: Report of two cases. *Neurosurgery* 1998; **42**:1390–1393.

Tubbs RS, Bui CJ, Rice WC, Loukas M, Naftel RP, Holcombe MP, Oakes WJ. Critical analysis of the Chiari malformation Type I found in children with lipomyelomeningocele. *J Neurosurg* 2007; **106**:196–200.

Tubbs S, Winters RG, Naftel RP, Acharya VK, Conklin M, Shoja MM, Loukas M, Oakes WJ. Predicting orthopedic involvement in patients with lipomyelomeningoceles. *Child's Nerv Syst* 2007; **23**:835–838.

Van Calenbergh F, Vanvolsem S, Verpoorten C, *et al.* Results after surgery for lumbosacral lipoma: The significance of early and late worsening. *Child's Nerv Syst* 1999; **15**:439–443.

Wood BP, Harwood-Nash DC, Berger P, *et al.* Intradural spinal lipoma of the cervical cord. *AJR* 1985; **145**:174–176.

Wu HY, Kogan BA, Baskin LS, *et al.* Long-term benefits of early neurosurgery for lipomyelomeningocele. *J Urol* 1998; **160**:511–514.

Xenos C, Sgouros S, Walsh R, *et al.* Spinal lipomas in children. *Pediatr Neurosurg* 2000; **32**:295–307.

## Chapter 8

# Meningocele

---

### Definition

Meningocele is defined as herniation of only the meninges through a defective posterior neural arch. As the cystic mass in meningocele contains non-neural elements, it is called a *meningocele* and not a *myelomeningocele*. From the clinical point of view, meningocele definitely has a better prognosis with near normal neurological outcome than its open dysraphic counterpart, myelomeningocele. However, meningocele are less frequent than myelomeningocele.

### Incidence

- 1 to 2 per 1000 live births
- Account for 10% of all spinal dysraphism
- Female preponderance is observed

### Location

The most common location of meningocele is the lower lumbar or lumbosacral region, followed by cervical and then the thoracic level.

The following image shows a very large thoracic meningocele in a completely normal child. Nonetheless, the size and appearance of the lesion compelled the parents of this child to abandon her, presuming that they will have to raise a severely handicapped individual.

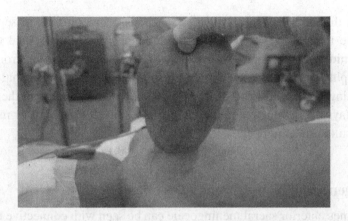

In the image below, the meningocele is lumbar and has an appearance suggestive of being a lipomeningocele. Surgical exploration and/or radiological studies clarify the diagnosis.

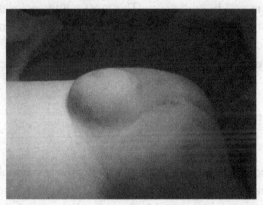

## Genetics

Almost all meningocele are sporadic in occurrence and only a few cases reported autosomal dominant pattern of inheritance, with manifestations as a familial anterior sacral meningocele syndrome.

## Embryology

Meningocele are known to arise from limited dorsal myeloschisis, meaning incomplete fusion of the vertebral arches leading to herniation of meninges through the defect. As a result, the cutaneous ectoderm fails to separate from the neuroectoderm with maldevelopment of the myofascial tissue in the midline. Subsequently, a band of tissue or stalk extend from the dorsal spinal cord to the skin and thus result in tethering of the spinal cord. Depending on the presence of hydromyelia, the central canal in the stalk either stays open, which would then result in a myelocystocele, or regress with resultant meningocele.

## Pathogenesis of Non-dysraphic Meningocele

Sometimes anterior sacral meningocele can be seen with connective tissue disorders like Marfan syndrome. These meningoceles are seen in non-dysraphic spinal column and associated commonly with neurofibromatosis and Marfan syndrome. These meningoceles arise due to congenital meso-dermal dysplasia and bony defects. The most common location for non-dysraphic meningoceles is the thoracic spine and they are termed lateral or anterolateral meningoceles. On the contrary, meningocele seen with spinal dysraphism is located mostly in the lumbar or lumbosacral region.

## Variants of Meningocele

### Myelocystocele

This is described as a "cyst within cyst" with the inner sac containing a cyst which communicates with the central canal and the outer sac communicates with the spinal arachnoid space. Myelocystocele is associated more often with Chiari malformation and hydrocephalus than meningocele.

### Currarino triad and anterior sacral meningocele (ASM)

Anterior sacral meningocele is a rare variant which is associated with anterior sacral defects and is part of the Currarino triad, which is a triad of anorectal anomalies combined with anterior sacral bony defect and associated anterior sacral meningocele. The clinical presentation of this rare clinical entity is usually in adulthood and presents mostly with gastrointestinal complaints of constipation and abdominal pain.

## Antenatal Diagnosis

Spina bifida can be diagnosed by fetal ultrasound during the second trimester. However, it is difficult to differentiate between myelomeningocele and simple meningocele. As the outcome of meningocele is extremely favorable as compared to myelomeningocele, fetal MRI should be undertaken for confirmation of meningocele if termination of pregnancy is contemplated.

## Clinical Presentations

As there is no neural element involved, children are born with near normal neurological examinations. However, secondary neurological deterioration may develop from concurrent spinal pathologies, as seen in 90% cases with meningocele. The presence of such pathologies that may lead to late onset of neurological symptoms. These concurrent pathologies are briefly mentioned here.

- Thickened filum terminale
- Tethered cord syndrome
- Diastematomyelia
- Hydromyelia/Syringomyelia

The most common of the abovementioned pathologies is thickened filum terminale, which can present clinically as tethered cord syndrome. Evaluation with MRI is recommended for such obscure lesion.

## Surgery

Follow the rules common to all other NTD. Protect viable tissue with adequate dural plane and remove the abnormal tissue. In the case of meningoceles the abnormal central nervous system within the sac is minimal, if any.

## Suggested Readings

Arts MP, de Jong TH. Thoracic meningocele, meningomyelocele or myelocystocele? Diagnostic difficulties, consequent implications and treatment. *Pediatr Neurosurg* 2004; **40**(2):75–79.

126                                      *Neural Tube Defects*

Erşahin Y, Barçin E, Mutluer S. Is meningocele really an isolated lesion? *Child's Nerv Syst* 2001; **17**(8):487–490.

Gardner P, Albright L. Hereditary anterior sacral meningocele. *J Neurosurg* 2006; **104**:138–142.

Salomão JF, Cavalheiro S, Matushita H, Leibinger RD, Bellas AR, Vanazzi E, de Souza LA, Nardi AG. Cystic spinal dysraphism of the cervical and upper thoracic region. *Child's Nerv Syst* 2006; **22**:224–234.

Chapter 9

# Hemimyelomeningocele

## Definition

Hemimyelomeningocele is considered under the terminology of complex spinal dysraphism and is a rare pathology which can lead to confusion and delay in diagnosis. Hemimyelomeningocele is defined as presence of myelomeningocele in one of the hemicords of the diastematomyelia.

## Incidence

The true incidence and exact embryological origin of hemimyelomeningocele is not known yet. However, the incidence is reported to be 2–10% of cases in children with concurrent presence of split cord malformation.

## Embryology

Although the exact mechanism is not known yet, a possible theory of origin of hemimyelomeningocele is explained as follows. Gastrulation defects lead to formation of split notochord and subsequent formation of hemicords. From the presence of individual central canal, it can be deduced that each hemicord undergoes neurulation process independently. The persistence of the endomesenchymal tracts may interfere with the normal closure of the neural tube and induce secondary opening of neural tube in the hemicord as seen in myelomeningocele cases.

## Clinical Presentation

The neurological deficits are seen on the side of hemicord with the open neural tube or myelomeningocele described as follows:

- Less severe neurological deficits as compared to conventional MMCL.
- Asymmetrical examination findings of legs with at times presence of completely normal function on one side.

127

- The child can have a completely normal bladder function and sphincter control.

I recall one of my patients who had an outstanding clinical outcome following closure of lower lumbar myelomeningocele. We believed that it was an extraordinary case until the child's clinical evolution, equinovarus in his case, prompted an MRI to be taken and only then it was elucidated that the normal hemicord was responsible for the child's outcome as well as for its clinical deterioration because of tethering.

## Suggested Reading

Jans L, Vlummens P, Van Damme S, Verstraete K, Abernethy L. Hemimyelomeningocele: A rare and complex spinal dysraphism. *JBR-BTR* 2008; **91**(5):198–199.

# Chapter 10

# Diastematomyelia

## Definition

Diastematomyelia, also called split cord malformation (SCM), belongs to the group of spinal dysraphism, where the spinal cord is split over a variable distance into two neural tubes or hemicords with presence of an osseous or osseo-cartilaginous septum in between the two cord segments.

## Historical Review

The oldest specimen of diastematomyelia, dating back to early 18th century, was recovered in the tomb of a 20-year-old man in Negev Desert, Israel. The mummy showed the presence of butterfly vertebrae and osseous spur. The term *diastematomyelia* was first used by French pathologist, Ollivier d'Angers in 1837, from the Greek words *"diastema"* (cleft) and *"myelos"* (spinal cord).

Herren and Edwards collected 43 cases of split cord malformation from autopsy specimens at the end of the 19th century. Finally it was a surgeon by the name of Hamby who was the first to operate on diastematomyelia in 1950. The advent of CT in 1970 and later the MRI in the 1980 helped diagnose and understand diastematomyelia better.

## Incidence

- 3–20% of patients with tethered cord harbor diastematomyelia
- More common in females

### Geographical incidence

Low rates of diastematomyelia have been reported in Japan whereas high incidence has been reported in India and Turkey.

## Age of Presentation

Four years on average is the usual age of presentation. However, there is a bimodal age of distribution with the first peak in childhood between two and five years and the second peak at 12–16 years during period of rapid growth.

## Genetic Basis

Most diastematomyelia cases are sporadic in nature with a few familial cases reported in the literature indicating possible recessive trait of inheritance.

## Embryology

### Persistence of accessory neurenteric canal (ANC)

The universally accepted theory of origin of diastematomyelia is that the primary defect originates from either formation or persistence of the accessory neurenteric canal between the yolk sac and the amnion. This connection is filled with mesenchyme, with the resultant formation of an endomesenchymal tract that splits or divides the notochord and the developing neural tube. The result is a split cord or presence of two hemicords. We present here a historical review of the embryogenesis of this unique spinal dysraphic state.

### Bremmer *et al.* theory

Bremmer *et al.* proposed the following theory: The primitive neurenteric canal is a communication between the amnion, an ectodermal derivative, and the yolk sac, an endodermal derivative. This neurenteric cyst disappears almost immediately after its formation in a spontaneous manner. After the physiological disappearance of neurenteric canal, a second endo–ectodermal communication develops and it is called the accessory neurenteric canal. It is the persistence of this accessory neurenteric canal which leads to the splitting of the notochord and subsequent formation of the two hemicords separated by a longitudinal septum.

### Pang *et al.* theory

Pang *et al.* acknowledged the theory put forth by Bremmer *et al.* and went on to elaborate further the pathogenesis of diastematomyelia and its accompanying pathologies. The persistence of the anterior part of this accessory neurenteric canal leads to anomalous development of the intestinal tract with malformations such as duplication of gut or formation of bands which result in intestinal malrotation. When the posterior part of the accessory neurenteric canal persists, the result is cutaneous malformations such as hypertrichosis, which is presence of tuft of coarse hair or aberrant vessels such as angiomas. Deeper skin lesions such as dermal sinus or the development of dermoid/epidermoid cyst have also been observed.

## Persistence of the intermediate part of ANC

However, it is the persistence of the intermediate part of this accessory neurenteric canal which has the most significant clinical implication as it results in division of the notochord and neural placode with sub-sequent development of split cord malformation or diastematomyelia. The endomesenchymal tract described earlier retains the potential to differentiate into either an osseous/bony spur, remain fibrocartilaginous, or as a soft septum of fibrous tissue. Rarely the dividing septum develops into an aberrant tangle of blood vessels or even evolves into a complex arteriovenous malformation (AVM). Even rarer are the formation of a thick fibro-neurovascular stalk called "myelomeningocele manqué" or the formation of a dermal sinus tract.

## Clinical Classification Based on Embryologic Origin

### Type I

In this variant of diastematomyelia, there are two hemicords enclosed within their individual dural sheaths, separated by a purely osseous or rigid osseocartilaginous median septum. The embryology of type I split cord malformation (SCM) is explained by the fact that if the mesenchyme surrounding the ANC retains the precursor cells of meninges called the *meninx primitiva*, then this would lead to formation of two distinct dural sacs enclosing the two hemicords. At the same time, the two hemicords will be separated internally by an osseous or an osseocartilaginous spur arising from the differentiation of the retained cells of meninx primitiva, with the resultant formation of split spinal cord malformation of type I.

## Type II

In this variant of SCM, there is only one common dural sheath enclosing the two hemicords which are separated by a non-rigid median septum. This type of split cord malformation is also referred as *diplomyelia* in some old medical records. However, the term "type II" is universally accepted. Regarding the origin of type II SCM, it is explained as follows: If there is no persistence of cells from the meninx primitiva or the meningeal precursor cells, then the surrounding mesenchyme around the notochord induces the formation of a single dural sac enclosing the two hemicords with the remaining ANC, thus persisting as the non-rigid septum between the two hemicords.

## Classification Based on Radiological Diagnosis

This classification is based on the presence of the two following features:

- Number of dural tubes
- Nature of midline septum

## SCM type I

There is presence of double dural tubes separated by osseous or osseocartilaginous spur, with midline, vertical septum dividing the spinal cord into two equal compartments. However, paramedian nerve roots are absent.

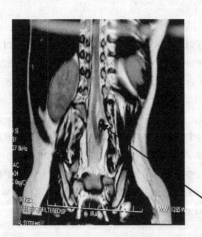

Septum splitting just a segment of the cord.

## SCM type II

There is presence of a single thecal sac enclosing the two hemicords, separated by non-rigid midline septum. Paramedian nerve roots are present in this variant.

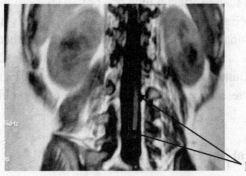

Hemicords

## Anatomical Localization of the Cleft

The position of cleft or the mid-sagittal septum is variable and can extend from one to ten vertebral segments. The following are location of the cleft in descending order of their incidence:

Lumbar: 47%
Thoracolumbar: 27%
Thoracic: 23%
Sacral or cervical: 1.5%
Multiple levels: <1%

### Pathophysiology of SCM

There are two separate entities:

- Intrinsic myelodysplasia
- Tethered cord syndrome

Direct compression of cord by the dividing septum or bony spur can lead to lower motor neuron type of neurological dysfunction. The clinical neurological complaints arise due to tethering of spinal cord, which leads to significant cord traction as the spur renders the cord inflexible. This is especially true during flexion–extension movements of the spine.

## Complex Spinal Dysraphism

The co-existence of SCM with MMCL is considered to be complex spinal dysraphism, with reported incidence of 15–39%. The embryological defect is considered to occur during the 3rd to 4th week of intrauterine life. The SCM malformation is seen to affect within one or two levels of the MMCL defect. These cases clinically present with a neurologically functional level discrepancy compared to the level of the defect. Another possible manifestation can be a progressive deterioration of the clinical picture after repair of the MMCL, and unexplained by the mere presence of tethered cord. This shows the relevance of evaluating a child of spina bifida with MRI of the spine.

### Secondary anatomical causes of tethering of conus medullaris in SCM

- Thickened filum
- Intradural lipoma
- Dermal sinus tract with or without dermoid cyst
- Myelomeningocele
- Hemimyelomeningocele

## Mechanisms of Cord Dysfunction by Tethering

i. *Mechanical factors*: The osseous or the fibrocartilaginous septum tethers the cord. Flexion and extension movements of the trunk are responsible for traction stress on the cord. Scoliosis and spinal canal stenosis further aggravate the condition.

ii. *Vascular factors*: The hypothesis that compression of the anterior spinal artery by the spur can lead to ischemic damage to the cord is a possibility.

iii. *Anatomical factors*: At times there is asymmetrical division of the cord by an oblique septum into a major hemicord and a minor hemicord. Thus hypoplasia in one hemicord due to primary neurulation defect, such as hemineural placode ending in a myelocele sac, could account for the neuro-orthopedic deficit.

# Syndromes Associated with Split Cord Malformation

Split cord malformation is associated with the following syndromes:

## Klippel–Feil deformity and cervical diastematomyelia

The Klippel–Feil deformity is a craniocervical junction anomaly characterized by fusion of at least two cervical vertebrae. Clinically the child presents
with short neck, low hairline and restricted neck movements.

## Jarcho–Levin syndrome (spondylocostal dysplasia)

This is a rare syndrome consisting of multiple vertebral and rib anomalies,
resulting in early neonatal death from pulmonary insufficiency.

## Sacral agenesis syndrome

In this syndrome there is agenesis of derivatives of the caudal eminence
presenting with lower limb neurological deficits, gastrointestinal and
genitourinary abnormalities. Detailed description of this malformation will
be discussed in later sections.

## Inencephaly

An incompatible anomaly and also the rarest form of neural tube defect
characterized by raschisis or open spinal dysraphism involving the neck
and the occiput.

# Tumors Associated with Diastematomyelia

The following are the congenital tumors associated with diastematomyelia:

## Extrarenal Wilms tumor

Wilms tumor, or nephroblastoma, is the most common solid malignancy of
childhood arising from the embryonic renal tissue. Extrarenal Wilms tumor
is a rare entity associated with diastematomyelia and arises at sites like
retroperitoneum, inguinal region, sacrococcygeal and lumbosacral region.
Management of these tumors is the standard protocol for treating them.

**Teratoma**

Congenital tumors containing all three germ cell layers are called *teratoma* and they have a strong association with neural tube defects. Sacrococcygeal site is a common location for these tumors. Prognosis of these congenital tumors is good with rare instances of malignant degeneration.

**Cerebellar heterotopias**

A rare cerebellar migrational disorder is at times associated with split cord malformations.

**Neurenteric cyst**

Classified as a type of neural tube defect, neurenteric cyst is a rare entity associated with abnormal notochordal development. Most common location is the cervical region with case reports citing the presence of this entity in the lower lumbar and lumbosacral region.

**Associated Visceral Anomalies**

Diastematomyelia is also accompanied at times by the following visceral malformations:

- Situs inversus totalis
- Uterus didelphis
- Bifid scrotum
- Ureteral duplication
- Duplication of renal pelvis
- Anomalous origin of renal artery
- Intestinal malrotation and duplication of gut

**Antenatal Diagnosis of Split Cord Malformation**

Antenatal diagnosis of split cord malformation is difficult and there are only 16 cases reported so far in the literature, as diagnosed during antenatal period by ultrasonography. The most striking feature in the detection of diastematomyelia is an echogenic focus in the posterior aspect of the spine with a widening of the interpedicular vertebral space. This is a highly specific sign of antenatal diagnosis of diastematomyelia. There is anteroposterior narrowing of vertebral bodies with increase in interpedicular distance along with narrow disc spaces with occasional fusion of adjacent lamina. Presence of septum between hemicords is osseous in 75% of cases and fibrous in 25% of cases.

## Clinical Manifestations

Diastematomyelia usually manifests in childhood with only few cases of presentations of split cord malformation in adults are reported. The differences between the manifestations in both groups are:

- Adult onset is more abrupt in clinical presentation.
- Adult onset is usually preceded by some form of trauma or strenuous physical activity.
- Adult cases present most commonly with sensory complaints of pain and paresthesias.
- Adult onset neurological profile is usually progressive and deficits do not recover completely, indicating the irreversibility of adult onset neurological deficits.

### Children with SCM

Children with SCM are grouped into two categories:

1. Group I — Cutaneous markers in asymptomatic children
2. Group II — Symptoms of neuro-orthopedic and urological system

**1. Group I**: Children with cutaneous markers are usually asymptomatic but can have subtle signs of neurological dysfunction like mild atrophy of leg muscles, presence of scoliosis, or dulling of the superficial reflexes. At times the only abnormality may be detected by urodynamic studies as an incidental finding during evaluation of the renal functions.

Common cutaneous markers which indicate underlying split cord malformations include:

- Hypertrichosis
- Dermal sinus with intraspinal dermoid cyst
- Capillary hemangioma
- Rare subcutaneous lipoma

Among the cutaneous markers accompanying split cord malformation, hypertrichosis is the most common, occurring with an incidence of 50–60% of cases. The incidence of this cutaneous marker is followed by capillary hemangioma. However, the combined presence of hairy patch with underlying hemangioma is not uncommon. The rare forms of cutaneous signs associated with split cord malformation are dermal sinus or dermoid cyst.

Etiology of the cutaneous markers can be deduced from the fact that the anomalous development of the underlying neural tube as a direct effect of the endomesenchymal tract leads to secondary maldevelopment of the surface ectoderm. This is manifested as various cutaneous markers.

2. **Group II**: In this group, the children present with various complaints suggestive of tethered cord syndrome. Usually the children in this group are asymptomatic at birth and continued to remain so for some time. These children become symptomatic insidiously but abrupt clinical presentations have been known to occur after strenuous exercises like ballet dancing or gymnastics. Some children may present without antecedent trauma or physical activity and coincide with phases of rapid growth.

   i. *Neurological symptoms*: Common complaints pertaining to the neurological dysfunction include pain in the lower back or legs. Paresthesias and dysthesias are often described by children as fuzzy feeling of legs or the child may appear irritable and has temper tantrums. The following are characteristics of pain seen in SCM:

      **Quality**: The pain is usually described as sharp and well-localized.
      **Distribution**: The pain usually follows dermatomal pattern which is indicative of root or plexus localization and is compatible with the spinal segment of pointing towards the location of SCM.
      **Associated features**: Pain is accompanied with paresthesias and dysthesias, described by the child as a tingling feeling in the legs or feeling of "pins and needles on the skin".
      **Sensory loss**: Occasionally sensory loss is apparent and is described by the child as numbness in the legs and with presence of recurrent injuries.
      **Motor complaint**: Weakness in leg is usually asymmetrical and is manifested as dragging of leg or limping.

**On examination**: Ask the child to hop. Usually subtle weakness of legs can be detected by asking the child to hop on one foot. The following are the neurological profile described:

- Inability to walk on heels — weakness of dorsiflexors with spinal segment at L5.
- Inability to walk on toes — weakness of plantar flexors with spinal segment at S1.
- Poor muscle tone especially inability to sit — truncal hypotonia, a manifestation of split cord malformation localized to cervical region.

**Gait**: Gait instability or deterioration is an early sign. The child is described as being clumsy with frequent falls and injuries.

**Autonomic dysfunction (sympathetic dystrophy)**: Autonomic disturbances are seen in 15% of children with diastematomyelia and are described as having thin, shiny and hairless skin. There is presence of anhydrosis, i.e. decreased sweating and dependant rubor in legs. Thickening and fissuring of toe nails are also observed. The clinical implication of development of sympathetic dystrophy can lead to injuries and ulceration of skin with subsequent formation of chronic trophic ulcer. In very rare cases the infection can spread to the phalanges with resultant osteomyelitis and the most extreme symptom which is the autoamputation of toes (rarely seen in this modern medicine era).

ii. *Urological complaints*: The child can present with the following urological complaints:

- Polyuria (increased frequency of urination)
- Presence of urgency
- Repeated urinary tract infections
- Presence of urinary incontinence
- Nocturnal enuresis

These abovementioned conditions should prompt the treating physician to order diagnostic investigations to evaluate for neurogenic bladder. Rarely bowel complaints are seen in children with split cord malformation. The most common bowel complaint is constipation rather than incontinence.

iii. *Orthopedic complaints*: Orthopedic complaints in the form of deformity are usually observed and are asymmetrical. Worsening of head tilt or torticollis is seen in split cord malformation at cervical level. The most common deformity is progression of talipes deformity, which is walking on toes.

Older children can present with orthopedic complaints which are described as follows:

- Scoliosis is very commonly seen although kyphosis can also be present
- Sprengel's deformity (congenital elevation of shoulder blade on one side)
- Hip subluxation with limping gait
- Asymmetry of lower limbs
- Pes cavus, i.e. in-turned foot
- Pes varus and valgus

## Adult onset

In adults there is usually an abrupt onset with a precipitating event like strenuous exercise, trauma or prolonged lithotomy position, or in other words, activities with any degree of pronounced spine flexion. The most common symptom in adults is dysesthetic pain at perineal or perianal region, with occasional diffuse leg weakness. A phenomenon not seen in children is neurogenic claudication.

This is a sign where the patient gets painful cramps in legs after walking for a distance and is a classic sign of lumbar spinal cord dysfunction from traction or stenosis.

We were recently consulted on a 59-year-old woman suffering from tethered cord release in 2000, at that time presenting with decreasing ability to walk and bilateral lower extremity weakness. She experienced post-operative improvement in ambulation for 3–5 years, then began to have insidious onset of unsteady gait and falls, but they did not concern her enough to seek medical attention. She presented again to the hospital with one week of acute left leg radiculopathy and a herniated L5–S1 disc. On examination, she was found to display symptoms of tethered cord syndrome as well, with decreased rectal tone, quite profound weakness of all muscle groups in her left leg, and electric shock type of pain going down her back to her legs when flexing her neck, hips, and knees. She also had inability to hold her bowel and bladder for six months and was wearing diapers under her clothes.

## Radiological Investigations

MRI as a diagnostic investigation should be undertaken in evaluation of split cord malformation. Nonetheless, a plain X-ray can also be informative. The following are radiological signs of diastematomyelia seen in an X-ray spine.

Widening of the spinal canal with increase in interpedicular distance is perhaps the most diagnostic sign seen in an X-ray spine. This picture is also seen in spinal tumors but they have erosion associated with tumors, which is never seen in split cord malformation. Other findings include incomplete fusion of vertebral bodies, presence of hemivertebra, decrease in height of vertebral bodies and scoliosis. The MRI image below reproduces some of the findings that can be seen with less sophisticated methods.

This classical image (axial cut with arrow pointing towards the septum) corresponds to the 59-year-old patient whose case was described earlier.

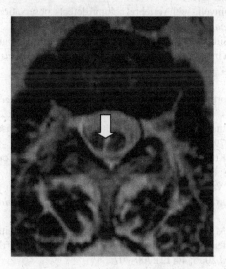

## Surgery

The objective of the surgery is to completely remove the spur. Properly performed, there should be no complications.

The pre-operative and post-operative images below are explicit.

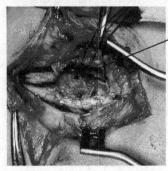
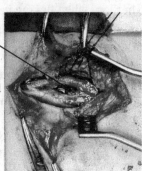

Septum before and after

The hemicords are observed without central roots. There was a common dural sheet.

## Suggested Readings

Bedru A, Mune T, Assefa G, Meseret S. Diastematomyelia: A case report with review of literatures. *Ethiop Med J* 2006; **44**(2):195–200.

Benedict Rilliet. The spine bifida, diastematomyelia. Springer, Milan 2006.

Bui CJ, Tubbs RS, Oakes WJ. Tethered cord syndrome in children: A review. *Neurosurg Focus* 2007; **23**(2):1–9.

Cowie TN. Diastematomyelia with vertebral column defects, observations on its radiological diagnosis. *Br J Radiol* 1951; **24**(279):156–160.

Dabra A, Gupta R, Sidhu R, Kochhar S, Kaur L, Singh J. Sonographic diagnosis of diastematomyelia in utero: A case report and literature review. *Australasian Radiology* 2001; **45**:222–224.

Dachling
P. Split cord malformation: Part II: Clinical syndrome. *Neurosurgery* 1992 September; **31**(3):481–500.

Eid K, Hochberg J, Saunders D. Skin abnormalities of the back in diastematomyelia. *Plast Reconstr Surg* 1979; **63**(4):534–539.

Erşahin Y, Mutluer S, Kocaman S, Demirtaş E. Split spinal cord malformations in children *J Neurosurg* 1998; **88**:57–65.

Gan YC, Sgouros S, Walsh AR, Hockley AD. Diastematomyelia in children: Treatment outcome and natural history of associated syringomyelia. *Child's Nerv Syst* 2007; **23**:515–519.

Grossmann, Maeder I-M, Dollfus P. Treatise on the spinal marrow and its diseases (anatomy, functions and general considerations on its diseases) by Ollivier d'Angers CP (1796–1845) *Spinal Cord* 2006; **44**(12):700-707.

Kondo A, Kamihira O, Ozawa H. Neural tube defects: Prevalence, etiology and prevention. *Int J Urol* 2009; **16**(1):49-57.

Izci Y, Gonul M, Gonul E. The diagnostic value of skin lesions in split cord malformations. *J Clin Neurosci* 2007; **14**:860–863.

Lewandrowski KU, Rachlin JR, Glazer PA. Diastematomyelia presenting as progressive weakness in an adult after spinal fusion for adolescent idiopathic scoliosis. *Spine J* 2004; **4**(1):116–119.

Matson DD, Woods RP, Campbell JB, Ingraham FD. Diastematomyelia (congenital clefts of the spinal cord), diagnosis and surgical treatment. *Pediatrics* 1950; **6**(1):98–112.

Miller A, Guille JT, Bowen JR. Evaluation and treatment of diastematomyelia. *J Bone Joint Surg Am* 1993; **75**(9):1308–1317.

Oliver CP. Traite des Maladies de la Moelle Epiniere. 3rd ed, Vol. 1. Paris, Mequignon-marvis, 1837.

Pang D. Split cord malformation: Part II: Clinical syndrome. *Neurosurgery* 1992; **31**(3):481–500.

Pang D, Dias MS, Ahab-Barmada M. Split cord malformation: Part I: A unified theory of embryogenesis for double spinal cord malformations. *Neurosurgery* 1992; **31**(3):451–480.

Proctor MR, Scott RM. Long-term outcome for patients with split cord malformation. *Neurosurg Focus* 2001; **10**(1):e5.

Rossi A, Cama A, Piatelli G, Ravegnani M, Biancheri R, Tortori-Donati P. Spinal dysraphism: MR imaging rationale. *J Neuroradiol* 2004; **31**(1):3–24.

Schijman E. Split spinal cord malformations: Report of 22 cases and review of the literature. *Child's Nerv Syst* 2003; **19**:96–103.

Sinha S, Agarwal D, Mahapatra AK. Split cord malformations: An experience of 203 cases. *Child's Nerv Syst* 2006; **22**:3–7.

Sonigo-Cohen P, Schmit P, Zerah M, Chat L, Simon I, Aubry MC, Gonzales M, Pierre-Kahn A, Brunelle F. Prenatal diagnosis of diastematomyelia. *Child's Nerv Syst* 2003; **19**(7–8):555–560.

Uzumcugil A, Cil A, Yazici M. The efficacy of convex hemiepiphysiodesis in patients with iatrogenic posterior element deficiency resulting from diastematomyelia excision. *Spine* 2003; **28**(8):799–805.

## Chapter 11

# Terminal Myelocystocele

## Definition

The term myelocystocele was first introduced by Lassman *et al.* who observed the presence of dilatation of the terminal end of the central canal, often called the fifth ventricle, severe enough to be herniated through a posterior defect in the neural arch, forming a visible cystic bulge or mass at the lower back. The authors did acknowledge the much less severity in neurological dysfunction seen with terminal myelocystocele as compared to the more obvious exposed neural placode in MMCL and thus rightly named this defect as *spina bifida cystica minor* or *myelocystomeningocele*.

True to its name, this pathology is seen in the lumbar region in majority of cases, although it has the potential to arise at any spinal level. Thus terminal myelocystocele adds to the list of fluctuant lumbosacral mass present at birth.

## Non-terminal myelocystocele

Non-terminal myelocystocele is even rarer than its terminal counterpart and is often misdiagnosed as meningocele. This clinical entity is described by the presence of posterior spinal defect, a CSF-filled cyst, an enlarged dural sheath (meningocele) and dorsal fat continuous with the subcutaneous fat. The non-terminal myelocystocele is further divided into two varieties: type I, called *myelocystocele manqué*, which is characterized by the presence of a transversing fibroneurovascular stalk; and type II, where the focal hydromyelia has displaced the posterior spinal wall into the meningocele sac. Compared to the terminal variety, the non-terminal myelocystocele has a better prognosis and clinical outcome.

## Epidemiology

**Incidence**: Very rare anomaly and accounts for 4–8% of occult spinal dysraphism.

**Genetics**: Sporadic in nature with no familial pattern being reported in literature.

**Etiology**: Exact mechanism not known.

**Teratogens**: Hydantoin/loperamide (antidiarrheals)/retinoic acid have been implicated as causative factors. In fact in experimental studies, retinoic acid has been shown to produce myelocystocele in golden hamsters.

## Theories Explaining Origin of Terminal Myelocystocele

Terminal myelocystocele is a congenital anomaly arising from the abnormalities of the caudal cell mass. The caudal cell mass is formed from the fusion of the notochord and neural epithelium. Precursors of caudal spinal cord, i.e. the sacral and the coccygeal segments along the hindgut and the embryonic kidney have common origin from the caudal cell mass. Any aberration in the caudal cell mass will result in formation of myelocystocele, sacral dysgenesis, anorectal anomalies like imperforate anus or ambiguous genitalia and cloacal exstrophy (note that cloacal exstrophy can arise independent of myelocystocele). At 38 days the caudal neural tube undergoes retrogressive differentiation to form the distal conus medullaris, filum terminale and the ventricular terminalis, or the 5th ventricle.

### McLone and Naidich theory

For unknown reasons the CSF is unable to exit with resultant accumulation of CSF and subsequent dilation of terminal ventricle. This disrupts the dorsal mesenchyme but not the surface ectoderm, which explains the spina bifida with skin-covered lesion. Thus spinal defects occur secondary to distension followed by rupture of the terminal ventricle, leading to a skin-covered spinal defect. Continued growth of the ventriculus terminalis due to accumulation of CSF causes distension of the distal thecal sac, forming a meningocele and this prevents the normal ascent of the cord, resulting in a tethered cord syndrome which is known to cause late-onset neurological deficit in these patients. The abnormality in CSF dynamics is local and thus is rarely associated with hydrocephalus and children with terminal myelocystocele have normal intellectual development. There is free communication between the myelocystocele and the central canal and between the meningocele and the subarachnoid space; however, there is no communication between the myelocystocele and the meningocele.

## Clinical Presentation

### Examination of the lumbosacral mass and its differentials

- Skin covered (always).
- Overlying skin normal but may have stigmata of occult spinal dysraphism such as hemangioma, nevus, hypertrichosis, skin dimple, and dermal sinus.
- Fluctuation test positive.
- Obliteration of intergluteal cleft (in lipomyelomeningocele there is most of the time distortion of the intergluteal cleft).

### Examination findings

Clinical presentation is variable ranging from normal neurological examination at birth to complex pathological issues. The following are types of presentations:

  i. Foot deformity — varus or valgus deformity
 ii. Limb asymmetry
iii. Spinal deformity

- Scoliosis
- Sacral dysgenesis

 iv. Neurological deficits

- Motor/sensory
- Sphincter disturbances

  v. Neurologically intact

### Associated visceral anomalies

Terminal myelocystocele is often a part of OEIS complex which include the following anomalies:

- **O**mphalocele

- Exstrophy of bladder
- Imperforate anus
- Spinal dysraphism

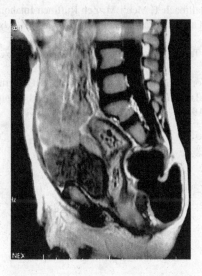

## Diagnostic Investigation

MRI is the diagnostic procedure of choice.

- It reveals the presence of dilated ventriculus terminalis with a trumpet-like flare.
- Meningocele is usually present beside or around the myelocele and herniates into the subcutaneous tissue.

## Management

Late onset of neurological deterioration occurs from tethering of cord and hydromyelic dilatation. Therefore, prophylactic early untethering of cord is recommended as terminal myelocystocele carries a favorable prognosis.

## Suggested Readings

Cartmill M, Jaspan T, Punt J. Terminal myelocystocele: An unusual presentation. *Pediatr Neurosurg* 2000; **32**:83–85.

Choi JS, McComb G. Long-term outcome of terminal myelocystocele patients. *Pediatr Neurosurg* 2000; **32**:86–91.

Jaiswal AK, Mahapatra AK. Terminal myelocystocele. *J Clin Neurosci* 2005; **12**(3), 249–252.

Kolble N, Huisman T, Stallmach T, Meuli M, Zen Ruffinen Imahorns F, Zimmermann R. Prenatal diagnosis of a fetus with lumbar myelocystocele. *Ultrasound Obstet Gynaecol* 2001; **18**:536–539.

Natarajan Muthukumar. Terminal and nonterminal myelocystoceles. *J Neurosurg* 2007; **107**(2):87–97.

Scott H, Meyer SH, Morris GF, Pretorius DH, James HE. Terminal myelocystocele: Important differential diagnosis in the prenatal assessment of spina bifida. *J Ultrasound Med* 1998; **17**:193–197.

## Chapter 12

# Caudal Regression Syndrome

## Definition

The maldevelopment of caudal eminence in an embryo before the fourth week of gestation due to abnormal development of the caudal mesoderm is called *caudal regression syndrome* (CRS). The spectrum of defects range from the most severe aspect called *sirenomelia* or *mermaid syndrome* to minor anomalies of bony defect compatible with prolonged life.

## Historical Review

Duhamel was the first to introduce the term caudal regression syndrome after his descriptive analysis of abnormal development of the caudal mesoderm of embryo before the fourth week of gestation.

## Incidence

- Rare anomaly with expected incidence of 1 in 60,000 births
- Male to female ratio is 2.7:1
- Diabetes is a known risk factor with 16% incidence of caudal regression syndrome seen in women with gestational diabetes
- Teratogens like vitamin A and other drugs like minoxidil may also play a role in pathogenesis

## Molecular Genetics and Genetic Counseling

Most cases of CRS are sporadic and the few familial cases reported in the literature seems to display an X-linked dominant pattern of inheritance. The HOMEOBOX gene has been detected as the cause in autosomal dominant sacral agenesis syndrome. With risk factors like maternal diabetes or presence of familial cases, the recurrence risk is less than 5%.

## Embryology

CRS is a neural tube defect that occurs before 28 days of gestation with maldevelopment of caudal eminence resulting secondarily from abnormal para-axial mesoderm. The most severe form of CRS is called sirenomelia, or mermaid syndrome, with fused lower limbs and multiple associated visceral anomalies. Sirenomelia arises from placental insufficiency or a result of vasoconstriction of placental circulation leading to decreased vascular supply to the fetus. Teratogens like cocaine have also been implicated in the pathogenesis of sirenomelia.

The associated visceral anomalies seen in caudal regression syndrome can be explained by the fact that during the process of secondary neurulation, the caudal end of the neural tube and the notochord blend into a caudal cell mass called *caudal eminence*, which lies adjacent to the developing hindgut and mesonephros. This juxtaposition of developing hindgut/genitourinary/notochord/neural structures within the tail fold accounts for caudal regression syndrome's common association with visceral and vertebral anomalies.

## Association of Diabetes and Caudal Regression Syndrome

Incidence of CRS in children born to diabetic mothers is 16–22%. Diabetes acts as a teratogen during the third to seventh week of organogenesis, as hyperglycemia-induced glycosylation of proteins is the cause of alteration of genes that control extracellular matrix component. In fact, Greene *et al.* have deduced a risk percentage for maternal diabetes and glucose control:

- HbA1C < 6.9% normal — no risk of congenital anomaly
- HbA1C < 9.3% — 3% risk of congenital malformation
- HbA1C < 14.4% — 40% risk of congenital malformation

## Pathology of Caudal Regression Syndrome

| Primary Structural Defect | Secondary Effects |
| --- | --- |
| Agenesis or incomplete development of lower lumbosacral vertebrae | Disruption of appropriate length of spinal cord and development of scoliosis |
| Spinal cord disruption | Neurological deficits such as bladder and bowel incontinence, motor and sensory deficits |
| Lower limb involvement | Joint contractures and dislocation, popliteal webs |

## Associated Visceral Anomalies in Caudal Regression Syndrome

| System Involved | Defects |
| --- | --- |
| Musculoskeletal | 1. Club foot or talipes equinovarus<br>2. Pelvic deformity with dislocation of hip joint<br>3. Flexion contractures of hip/knee joint<br>4. Scoliosis/kyphoscoliosis<br>5. Absent fibula/radii/ribs<br>6. Syndactyly/polydactyly<br>7. Pierre Robin Syndrome |
| Gastrointestinal System | 1. Anorectal malformation like imperforate anus<br>2. Tracheo-esophageal fistula<br>3. Abdominal wall defects like inguinal hernia<br>4. Intestinal obstruction from malrotation of gut/duodenal or colonic atresia |
| Genitourinary System | 1. Renal agenesis, dysplasia or fusion<br>2. Hydronephrosis<br>3. Vesicoureteric reflux<br>4. Ectopic ureter<br>5. Absent bladder<br>6. Vesical or cloacal exstrophy<br>7. Rectovaginal or rectourethral fistula<br>8. Hypospadias |

## Pathogenesis of Clinical Picture in CRS

The abnormal migration of neural crest cells during primary neurulation is the cause of presence of heterotopic sensory ganglia in the sensory nerve roots. There is preservation of neurological function especially sensory function beyond the expected vertebral level, due to relative sparing of nerve roots in spite of absence or agenesis of vertebral segments, with increased plasticity among the remaining sensory ganglia which compensate by enlarging their territory of innervations.

## Classification

**Type I**: Partial or complete unilateral sacral agenesis.
**Type II**: Partial but bilateral and symmetrical sacral agenesis.
**Type III**: Total sacral agenesis with variable lumbar agenesis with the iliac bones articulating with the last lumbar vertebra.

**Type IV**: Complete sacral agenesis with the iliac bones fused together underneath the last lumbar vertebra.

## Prognosis

The level of spinal defect and the severity of associated malformations determine the prognosis. Some of the visceral defects are lethal like bilateral renal agenesis. Types I and II can reach community ambulatory ability but types III and IV have bad prognosis, mainly due to other systemic anomalies.

## Diagnosis

### Antenatal

*First trimester diagnosis* is difficult due to the presence of incomplete ossification of sacrum. However, the diagnosis can be determined using transvaginal sonogram with the following features:

- Short crown rump length
- Abnormal appearance of yolk sac
- Large nuchal translucency by the 16th week

*Second trimester diagnosis* as early as 22 weeks can be made by frog-like position of lower legs ("Buddha's position"), i.e. external rotation of hip joint with V-shape position of the femurs, with sudden interruption of the fetal spine.

### Postnatal evaluation

CT and plain X-ray help in delineating the osseous defect, with MRI being the investigation of choice as it helps to delineate not only the vertebral anomaly but also the associated visceral anomalies. Sometimes CRS is associated with progression of neurological symptoms, raising the possibility of tethered cord syndrome and MRI aids in the diagnosis of this condition. About 40–50% of anorectal malformations are known to be associated with caudal vertebral and spinal anomalies.

### Differential diagnosis

The following are conditions with the underlying common feature of sacral agenesis.

i. **Currarino's syndrome**: Sacral agenesis with anorectal and urogenital malformation with a presacral mass (like anterior meningocele or teratoma) presenting in an autosomal dominant pattern of inheritance.

ii. **VATER syndrome**: This condition may present with sacral agenesis along with anal stenosis, tracheo-esophageal fistula, absent radii with renal dysgenesis.

## Clinical Case

### Anterior myelomeningocele with caudal regression syndrome

*Case description*: With the help of a prenatal ultrasound, multiple anomalies were detected in this child *in utero*, including omphalocele, crossed fused ectopic kidney and vertebral anomalies. The child underwent multiple reparative bowel procedures. At two months of age the child presented with an episode of intractable vomiting and had dehydration. Ultrasonography performed detected a thickened filum terminale with tethered cord and anterior myelomeningocele.

Grade II vesicoureteral reflux and also MRI of thoracolumbar spine at 15 months of age showed the presence of a large lateral anterior thoracolumbar myelomeningocele underlying the liver and extending down to pelvis. Extensive holocord syrinx was noted along with lumbosacral dysraphism. Fused hemivertebra, fused ribs and scoliosis were also noted. X-ray pelvis showed deformity of iliac crest along with separation and asymmetry of pubic bones.

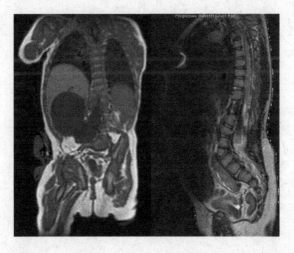

154                                   *Neural Tube Defects*

*Treatment plan*: At 17 months of age the child was operated for repair of anterior thoracolumbar myelomeningocele via the posterior approach. No post-operative complications were noted with the patient being discharged in stable clinical condition. During the follow-up, the child was in excellent clinical condition with full control of bladder and bowel. There was no sign of raised intracranial pressure and no significant tethering of spinal cord was detected either.

## Suggested Readings

Duhamel B. From the mermaid to anal imperforation: The syndrome of caudal regression. *Arch Dis Child* 1961; **36**:152–155.

Janet M, Stewart S, Stephen Stoll. Familial caudal regression anomalad and maternal diabetes. *J Med Genet* 1979; **16**:17–20.

Singh SK, Singh RD, Sharma A. Caudal regression syndrome — case report and review of literature. *Pediatr Surg Int* 2005; **21**:578–581.

Towfighi J, Housman C. Spinal cord abnormalities in caudal regression syndrome. *Acta Neuropathol* 1991; **81**:458–466.

# Chapter 13

# Dorsal Enteric Fistula

## Introduction

Dorsal enteric fistula can manifest as an isolated lesion or in combination with a wide array of malformations. This anomaly is handled by pediatric surgeons more than neurosurgeons due to its prominent bowel involvement. It belongs to those rare varieties of complex spinal dysraphism where a communication between the endoderm and ectoderm persists, resulting in its most severe form, a bowel ostium. In essence this syndrome is a combination of anterior and posterior spina bifida.

## Definition

A combination of anterior and posterior spinal defect in association with gastrointestinal anomaly, mostly in the form of fistulous connection between the developing gut and the neural tube is called *dorsal enteric fistula*. This is a defect of notochord integration and arises from splitting of the notochord. The split notochord syndrome had a variable expression. In its basic form, there is presence of a neural tube defect with persistence of an endo–ectodermal fistula opening at the dorsal aspect of the embryo. This means that there is a bowel ostium on the back of the patient. On rare occasions the urogenital system may also be involved.

## Embryology

The primary defect in split notochord syndrome is a persistent connection between the endoderm and dorsal ectoderm. During the third week of intrauterine development, the neurenteric canal is formed in the region of primitive knot and it establishes a communication between the amniotic cavity and the yolk sac (primitive intestinal cavity). This neurenteric canal is obliterated in a few days.

From these events taking place in the developing embryo, it is clear that the defect lies in the development of the notochord, neurenteric canal, and para-axial mesoderm forming the vertebrae.

The hypothesis of persistence of the neurenteric canal which gives rise to split notochord syndrome was put forth by Russian pathologist, A.O. Kovaleski in 1869. However, this theory failed to explain the variable location of the defect and the associated visceral anomalies.

The following are mentions of a few *theories* trying to explain the etiopathogenesis of split notochord syndrome:

Bremmer *et al.* in 1962 proposed the theory of existence of an accessory neurenteric canal. Bremmer stated that any connection or opening between the intestinal tract and the midline dorsal structures is due to complete or partial obliteration of this accessory canal. He also explained the variable level of involvement is secondary to the pathological migration of the Hensen's node which determines the dorsal axis of the embryo.

According to Saunders *et al.* in 1943, the split or duplication of the notochord is the primary underlying factor resulting in secondary herniation of the primitive gut through the defect in the notochord and subsequent adherence to the dorsal ectoderm.

Beardmore and Wigglesworth in 1958 suggested that adhesions between the endoderm (position of primitive streak) and the dorsal ectoderm (protochordal plate) could possibly lead to formation of an endo-mesenchymal tract which is nothing but an accessory neurenteric canal that could probably bisect the developing notochord. Thus, this theory which is a combination of the hypotheses mentioned above is currently the most accepted theory.

Recently, Stevenson *et al.* proposed the vascular insufficiency theory to explain the failure of closure of the neural tube. According to this theory, there is disruption in vascularization in the region of the neural folds which hinders the closure of neural tubes.

## Classification

Bentley and Smith classified the lesions into two broad categories:

1. **Visceral anomalies**: Fistula/sinuses/posterior enteric diverticulum/ posterior enteric cyst.

These include the posterior enteric remnants like mesenteric or posterior mediastinal duplications, diverticula or cysts, which are connected to the anterior aspect of the vertebral body by a fibrous stalk. Usually the vertebral body is bifid with rare presence of complete anterior and posterior spina bifida.

2. **CNS anomalies**: Anterior/posterior/combined spina bifida/diastematomyelia/diplomyelia/butterfly vertebrae.

### Histopathological examination of remnant of enteric origin

On histological examination, the presence of smooth muscles and enteric mucosa (columnar epithelium) can be seen. The appearance of the epithelium may vary depending on the gut adjacent to completely undifferentiated cells. Occasionally presence of bronchopulmonary tissues can be detected.

### Types of posterior enteric remnants

1. **Posterior enteric fistulae**: With the failure of obliteration of the embryonic endomesenchymal tract, there persists a connection starting from the gut, transversing through the mesentery or the mediastinum and the complete spina bifida which is usually a diastematomyelia or diplomyelia, with termination on the midline of the skin of the back.

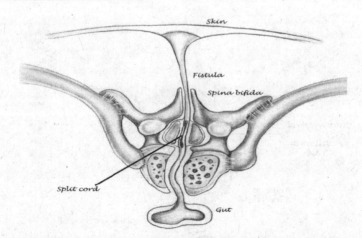

2. **Posterior enteric sinus**: Only the dorsal part of the embryonic fistula persists with a sinus tract running from the cutaneous or enteric tissues

which run forward to the skin of the back in the midline. There may be occassionally underlying posterior spina bifida.

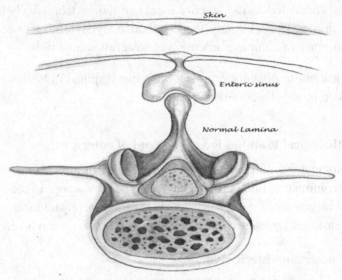

3. **Posterior enteric diverticula**: Only the ventral portion of the embryonic fistula remains and communicates with the gut. These cases are at risk for bowel strangulation or rotation. There may also be presence of underlying anterior or complete spina bifida.

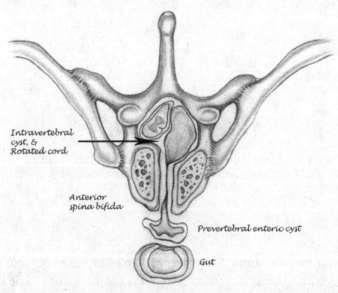

4. **Posterior enteric cyst**: Only an intermediate part of the embryonic fistula or diverticulum persists as a cyst, which may be pre-vertebral, vertebral or post-vertebral in position. Again spina bifida might be present, either of anterior or posterior type.

## Clinical features

**Site**: Most commonly involves the cervicothoracic spine with few reports of involvement of the lumbosacral spine.

**Neonatal presentations at birth**: Dorsal enteric fistula is the most severe condition. At birth, meconium is seen coming from the opening at the back. The main concern at this point is to undertake abdominal surgery to prevent further contamination and damage to the spinal cord.

**Early presentations**: Gastrointestinal obstruction or infection and meningitis.

**Delayed presentation**: Neurenteric cyst is infected with abscess.

Progressive neurological issues can arise with tethered cord or diastematomyelia.

## Management

- First step is to prevent contamination of the spinal cord
- Colostomy with excision of the fistula
- Closure of the spinal defect or untethering of cord to prevent further progression of neurological deterioration

## Suggested Readings

Agangi A, Paladini D, Bagolan P, Maruotti GM, Martinelli P. Split notochord syndrome variant: Prenatal findings and neonatal management. *Prenat Diagn* 2005; **25**:23–27.

Bentley JF, Smith JR. Developmental posterior enteric remnants and spinal malformations: The split notochord syndrome. *Arch Dis Child* 1960; **35**:76–86.

van Ramshorst GH, Lequin MH, Mancini GM, van de Ven CP. A case of split notochord syndrome: A child with a neurenteric fistula presenting with meningitis. *J Pediatr Surg* 2006; **41**:E19–E23.

Chapter 14

# Segmental Spinal Dysgenesis Syndrome

## Definition

Segmental spinal dysgenesis syndrome is a rare clinical condition characterized by the segmental dysgenesis of the vertebral column, with the most common location being the thoracolumbar or the lumbar spine. Scott *et al.* were the first to coin the term *segmental spinal dysgenesis syndrome* (SSD) and considered it to be distinct from other common lower vertebral anomalies like caudal regression syndrome. The highly pathognomonic clinical feature of SSD is the presence of segmental affection of the vertebral columns with normal cord present at the rostral end and near normal cord at the caudal end of the defect.

Closed spinal dysraphism and visceral anomalies including renal anomalies are often associated with SSD and may further aggravate the clinical condition. Such type of neural tube defects is considered by some to be part of more complex neural tube defects.

## Embryology

The embryogenesis of complex spinal dysraphism is considered to arise from defects during the gastrulation process. Gastrulation is the process by which the bilaminar embryonic disc gets converted into the trilaminar disc of ectoderm, endoderm and the intervening mesoderm. The process takes place approximately during the third week of gestation. Dias *et al.* hypothesized that complex dysraphic states arise because the mesodermal anlagen fail to integrate and instead remain separated and develop independently over various segments. The heterogeneity of expression of complex dysraphic states can range from complete split notochord syndrome, diastematomyelia, dermal sinus tract to caudal agenesis.

## Explaining SSD at the Molecular Level

Inappropriate apoptosis called *positional apoptosis* may underlie the etiopathogenesis of SSD. Apoptosis, also known as programmed cell death, plays an important role in normal embryogenesis. According to the present hypothesis, errors in signaling pathways lead to apoptosis of wrongly specified cells which are considered essential for normal embryogenesis, thus resulting in subsequent paucity of essential cells. This defective signaling probably underlies the paucity of chordamesodermal cells with resultant aplasia of a segment of spinal column, spinal cord and nerve roots.

## Pathogenesis

The clinical presentation depends on two factors: degree of dysfunction of the cord and functioning of the residual segment of the spinal cord. The presence of concurrent forms of occult spinal dysraphism further deteriorates the clinical condition. Commonly seen types of closed spinal dysraphism associated with SSD are split cord malformations, dermal sinus tract, terminal myelocystocele, spinal lipoma, and thick filum terminale.

## Clinical Presentation

The clinical presentation is variable, ranging from near normal neurological examination to presence of complete paraplegia.

i. *Neurological presentation*: The clinical presentation of this condition is marked by the presence of moderate to severe motor impairment of legs. Not all children born with SSD are paraplegic at birth. But they are vulnerable to further aggravation of their neurological status by concurrent presence of other closed spinal dysraphism like congenital instability of vertebral column or spinal canal stenosis. This factor should be kept in mind from the clinical outcome point of view as decompressive surgeries may not necessarily improve congenital paraplegia but would finitely halt the progressive deterioration of neurological functions.

ii. *Orthopedic complaints*: Lower limb deformities are a common accompaniment of this disorder with common clinical presentations such as flexion-adduction deformity of hips, flexion of knees and bilateral talipes equinovarus or club foot. The most severe form of deformity that can result from the abovementioned deformities is the "Buddha's position", i.e. complete paralysis of legs.

iii. *Urological complaints*:  All patients with SSD have neurogenic bladder, often complicated by vesicoureteral reflux and hydronephrosis with secondary urinary tract infections. Presence of renal anomalies further aggravate the urological complications. The types of congenital renal anomalies commonly seen with SSD are horseshoe kidney and renal ectopia.

## Diagnostic Investigations

The following investigations should be performed in a child with suspicion of SSD: X-ray spine and MRI spine for evaluation of spine, followed by urological workup which would include renal ultrasound and urodynamic studies.

The following are types of anomalies seen on radiological imaging:

**Vertebral body anomalies**: Aplasia or hypoplasia and hemivertebrae or butterfly vertebrae.

**Spine curvature defects**: Presence of moderate to severe kyphosis with the kyphotic apex called the gibbous which usually marks the level or segment of spinal pathology. At times there is presence of kyphoscoliosis. There is severe narrowing of the spinal canal at the level of the gibbous apex, even leading to spinal canal stenosis.

**Costal or rib anomalies**: When the SSD affects the thoracic spine, there is concomitant anomalous development of the ribs which are seen on the radiograph as bifid ribs, fused ribs or absent ribs.

## MRI imaging of the spine

The hallmark of this syndrome is the segmental involvement of the spinal cord. This means that there is presence of normal cord rostrally, followed by an abrupt change to a severely hypoplastic or indiscernible cord segment devoid of any nerve roots. Rarely the affected segment is only partially thinned with continuity of the central canal. Caudal to the affected segment, the spinal cord is thickened, bulky and is low-lying. The presence of spinal cord tissue below and above the affected abnormal segment is a pathognomonic feature of SSD. However, it should be noted that SSD-affected lower lumbar cord segment will have no further development of nervous tissue caudally.

## Associated Closed Spinal Dysraphism with SSD

MRI imaging of the spine aids in detecting associated closed spinal dysraphism like split cord malformation, dermal sinus, terminal myelo-cystocele, and thickened filum terminale. The dysraphic pathologies may be present above, at or below the affected cord segment.

## Treatment Planning

Decompressive surgery of spine and orthopedic management of kyphosis is the mainstay of treatment planning in SSD.

## Syndromes with Similar Presentation to SSD

The following are description of syndromes affecting the normal development of vertebral column which can be confused with SSD.

- Caudal regression syndrome
- Multiple vertebral segmentation disorder (Jarcho–Levin syndrome)
- Congenital vertebral displacement

The most distinct feature of this syndrome is the segmental affection of the cord with normal segments above and below the affected cord.

## Suggested Readings

Faciszewski T, Winter RB, Lonstein JE, Sane S, Erickson D. Segmental spinal dysgenesis: A disorder different from spinal agenesis. *J Bone Joint Surg [Am]* 1995; **77**:530–537.
Fondelli MP, Cama A, Rossi A, Piatelli GL, Tortori-Donati P. Segmental spinal dysgenesis: MRI findings in seven cases. *Neuroradiology* 1996; **38**(Suppl 2):89.
Hughes LO, McCarthy RE, Glasier CM. Segmental spinal dysgenesis: A report of three cases. *J Pediatr Orthop* 1998; **18**:227–232.

Scott RM, Wolpert SM, Bartoshesky LF, Zimbler S, Karlin L. Segmental spinal dysgenesis. *Neurosurgery* 1988; **22**:739–744.

Tortori-Donati P, Fondelli MP, Rossi A, Raybaud CA, Cama A, Capra V. Caudal regression syndrome — case report and review of literature. *Pediatr Surg Int* 2005 Jul; **21**(7):578–581.

# Chapter 15

# Neurenteric Cyst

## Definition

Neurenteric cyst has been described as a rare developmental anomaly considered as ectopic or displaced nest of cells derived from the endoderm. Neurenteric cyst is found at locations other than CNS and includes sites like mediastinum, abdomen and pelvis. In this narration we will describe the neurenteric cyst present only in the spinal cord.

## Demography

Neurenteric cyst accounts for 0.3–1.3% of spinal dysraphism. The most common site involved is the cervicothoracic junction followed by the craniocervical junction. However, a few case reports describing neurenteric cyst in the conus medullaris have been documented. Neurenteric cyst is virtually always present in the vertebral canal in an extramedullary location or outside the spinal cord and is ventral to the spinal cord.

## Wilkins and Odum Classification

Wilkins and Odum classified neurenteric cyst into the following three categories based on their histological picture of cyst wall and content of the cyst. The classification is as follows:

i. *Type A*: Cyst wall is lined with either gastrointestinal or respiratory epithelium consisting of pseudostratified columnar or cuboidal epithelium resting on basement membrane. Supranuclear vacuoles are observed (indicated by arrow). This is the most commonly seen neurenteric cyst.

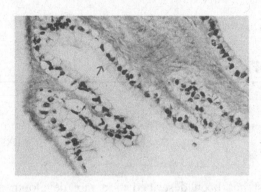

ii. *Type B*: Cyst wall is lined with glandular epithelium and it produces mucin or serous fluid.

iii. *Type C*: This is the most complex and also rarer form of neurenteric cyst containing ependymal or glial tissue.

## Embryology

Primary adhesion of the endoderm anterior to the notochord occurs with incomplete excalation process of the developing notochord. This results in persistence of neurenteric canal or accessory neurenteric canal with splitting of the notochord and displacement of the endodermal cells. This also explains the association of spinal cord anomalies with gastrointestinal anomalies seen with neurenteric cyst.

## Clinical Presentation

The clinical presentation and the severity of complaints depend on the location of the cyst and manifests as either myelopathy or radiculopathy.

- Neck pain and occipital headache
- Hemiparesis or paraparesis
- Chemical meningitis from cyst wall rupture
- Rarely the child may complain of dysesthetic pain

### Associated spinal and vertebral anomaly

- Split cord malformation
- Thick filum terminal

- Klippel–Feil deformity
- Hemivertebra

## Diagnostic Investigation

MRI is commonly used to diagnose this rare condition. However, the appearance of neurenteric cyst can be commonly confused with the more common arachnoid cyst. There are two radiological features used to identify a neurenteric cyst from an arachnoid cyst.

Neurenteric cysts are almost always present anterior to the spinal canal and usually have septae. However, the final conformation of neurenteric cyst is made after histopathological examination.

## Management

Neurenteric cyst should be treated surgically to prevent increasing neurological damage. During surgery there is the risk of cyst rupture and contamination with mucinous or serous content of the cyst with subsequent scarring and adhesion formation in the spinal cord. It is not infrequent that the symptoms may resolve by themselves.

## Suggested Readings

Lazareff JA, Hoil Parra JA. Intradural neurenteric cyst at the craniovertebral junction. *Child's Nerv Syst* 1995 Sep; **11**(9):536–538.

Lippman CR, Arginteanu M, Purohit D, Naidich TP, Camins MB. Intramedullary neurenteric cysts of the spine — case report and review of the literature. *J Neurosurg* 2001; **94**(2 Suppl):305–309.

Muzumdar D, Bhatt Y, Sheth J. Intramedullary cervical neurenteric cyst mimicking an abscess. *Pediatr Neurosurg* 2008; **44**(1):55–61.

Sheaufung S, Taufiq A, Nawawi O, Naicker MS, Waran V. Neurenteric cyst of the cervicothoracic junction: A rare cause of paraparesis in a paediatric patient. *J Clin Neurosci* 2009; **16**(4):579–581.

Tubbs RS, Salter EG, Oakes WJ. Neurenteric cyst — case report and a review of the potential dysembryology. *Clin Anat* 2006; **19**(7):667–669.

## Chapter 16

# Dermal Sinus

### Definition

A dermal sinus is an epithelium-lined tract that is usually considered a midline developmental anomaly along the neuraxis extending from the skin to a variable distance. Associated cutaneous anomalies seen with a dermal sinus such as hairy patch inside its orifice, hyperpigmented nevus and a capillary hemangioma have been reported in the literature.

The exact incidence is not known but it is considered a rare finding and is grouped under the umbrella term of *occult spinal dysraphism*.

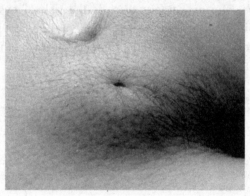

### Incidence

A reported incidence of 1 in 2500 live births is seen. The most frequent site of dorsal dermal sinus is the lumbar region (41%) followed by lumbosacral (23%), sacrococcygeal (13%), thoracic (10%) and lastly the cervical area (15%).

### Historical Review

Walker and Bucy were the first to coin the term *congenital dermal sinus* and reported the cases in association with development of meningitis.

## Embryogenesis

Incomplete separation of the cutaneous ectoderm from the underlying neuroectoderm has been implicated as the pathogenesis of dermal sinus tracts. Usually the cutaneous ectoderm and the neuroectoderm remain attached until the end of the neurulation process, which they then separate completely. Failure of this separation leads to dermal sinus tracts.

Dermal sinus tracts are variable and cases have been reported with extension of the tract to the dura mater and the underlying spinal cord to the more innocuous termination of the tract to the subcutaneous layers. Occasionally the tract terminates in the spina lipoma or is seen in association with open spina bifida.

## Clinical Manifestations

The most important clinical implication of the presence of dermal sinus tract is that the tract serves a route for infection, subsequently leading to meningitis or an intramedullary abscess with deleterious consequences. Thus the clinical manifestations of dermal sinus tract can be grouped as cutaneous, neurological and infectious.

### Associated conditions

Epidermoid or dermoid tumors are associated with dermal sinus. The figure below depicts an epidermoid tumor with the skin dimple at the extreme right of the tract.

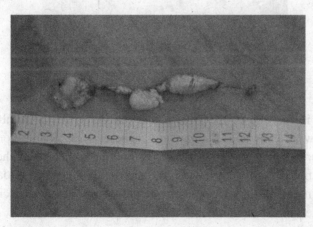

At times the cells proliferating within the dermal sinus contain excess of cholesterol crystals and can lead to chemical meningitis. The relevance of the latter should not be minimized because it can be fatal. Development of inclusion tumors or cysts can also contribute to neurological features.

### Neurological manifestations

Adult cases of dermal sinus presents with tethered cord syndrome or meningitis.

### Management

The objective of the surgery is to achieve complete excision of cyst with intradural exploration to identify potential sources of tethering of cord, and to prevent meningitis or the devastating intradural/intramedullary abscess. The pre-operative MRI should be informative enough to guide the surgical plan.

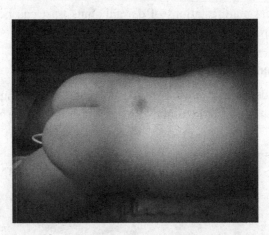

In the image above, the patient had the defect in the lumbar area, presented with fever and meningismus. There is reasonable concern to perform surgery in a patient with active meningitis. On the other hand, it can be argued that by removing the source of infection the danger of intradural/intramedullary abscess can be prevented. The final decision for surgery is left to the judgement of the treating team.

This image obtained during surgery demonstrates the link between the skin and the central nervous system.

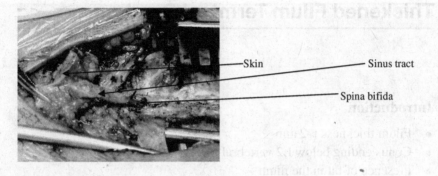

## Suggested Readings

Barkovich A, Edwards M, Cogen P. MR evaluation of spinal dermal sinus tracts in children. *AJNR* 1991; **12**:123–129.

Benzil D, Epstein M, Knuckey N. Intramedullary epidermoid associated with an intramedullary spinal abscess secondary to a dermal sinus. *Neurology* 1992; **30**:118–121.

Carrillo R, Carriera L, Prada J. Lateral congenital spinal dermal sinus. A new clinical entity. *Child's Nerv Syst* 1985; **1**:238–240.

Chen C, Lin K, Wang H. Dermoid cyst with dermal sinus tract complicated with spinal subdural abscess. *Pediatr Neurol* 1999; **20**:157–160.

Davis D, Cohen P, George R. Cutaneous stigmata of occult spinal dysraphism. *J Am Acad Dermatol* 1994; **31**:892–986.

Dev R, Husain M, Gupta A. MR of multiple intraspinal abscesses associated with congenital dermal sinus. *AJNR* 1997; **18**:742–743.

Hattori H, Higuchi Y, Tashiro Y. Dorsal dermal sinus and dermoid cysts in occult spinal dysraphism. *J Pediatr* 1999; **134**:793.

Hoil-Parra JA, Lazareff JA. Lumbar dermal sinus as a cause of intramedullary and subdural abscess — report of two cases. *Bol Med Hosp Infant Mex* 1993; **50**(5):341–346.

Kanev P, Park T. Dermoids and dermal sinus tracts of the spine. *Neurosurg Clin North Am* 1995; **6**:349–366.

Martinez-Lage J, Esteban J, Poza M. Congenital dermal sinus associated with an abscessed intramedullary epidermoid cyst in a child — case report and review of the literature. *Child's Nerv Syst* 1995; **11**:301–305.

McComb J. Disorders of the pediatric spine, congenital dermal sinus. Pang D (Ed), Raven Press, New York 1995, pp. 349–360.

Morandi X, Mercier P, Fournier H. Dermal sinus and intramedullary spinal cord abscess — report of two cases and review of the literature. *Child's Nerv Syst* 1999; **15**:202–206.

Wang K, Yang H, Oh C. Spinal congenital dermal sinus — experience of five cases over a period of ten years. *J Korean Med Sci* 1993; **8**:341–347.

## Chapter 17

# Thickened Filum Terminal Syndrome

### Introduction

- Filum thickness >2 mm
- Conus ending below L2 vertebral body
- Presence of fat in the filum

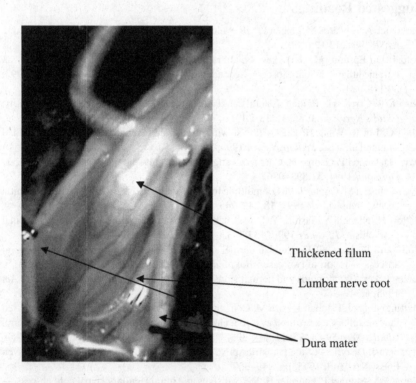

Thickened filum

Lumbar nerve root

Dura mater

The diagnosis is one of radiological finding with clinical correlation.

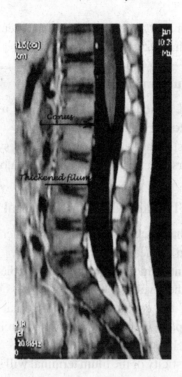

Thickened filum terminal is usually associated with low-lying conus which is below body of L2; however, normal lying conus can also be tethered with presence of a thickened filum terminal when it is called occult tethered cord syndrome.

Thickened filum terminal is a clinical entity where there is infiltration of the filum by fatty or fibrous tissue, subsequently resulting in tethered cord syndrome. The cord is descended and tethered in the great majority of cases. Nonetheless, the filum can be thickened, the patient symptomatic but the cord is not descended.

## Embryogenesis

### Defect in secondary neurulation

- Filum terminal is a cord-like extension of the terminal part of spinal cord which pierces the dura and anchors the cord to the coccyx.
- The filum develops during the retrogressive differentiation phase of the secondary neurulation process.

- Normal filum terminal contains ependymal and neuroglial cells and has a diameter of less than 0.5 mm.

### Origin of fat in the filum and its implication

- Faulty migration of mesodermal cells with their resultant retention in the filum give rise to fatty filum.
- Fatty filum is inelastic and leads to tethered cord syndrome.
- In rare cases, tumors like teratoma can be seen, along with fatty filum.

## Pathophysiology of Thickened Filum Terminal Syndrome

- It has been noted that there is a 7% increase in length of the vertebral canal during flexion of the spine.
- The dentate ligaments which anchor the cord to the adjoining vertebral canal terminate at the level of T12.
- The termination of the conus or the distal spinal cord segment is at level L1–L2 disc space with further continuation in the form of filum terminal, which anchors the conus to the coccyx.
- Any degree of inelasticity of the filum terminal will subsequently lead to traction of the cord, which will be most pronounced at the sacral level.
- As the sacral segment of the cord contains the bladder control center, this explains the phenomenon of intractable urinary complaints with minimal motor or sensory complaints in thickened filum terminal syndrome.

## Clinical Presentation

Clinically the patient may present with one of the following complaints:

- Urological
- Neurological
- Musculoskeletal and neurocutaneous markers

### Urological

- Most children present to the urologist with urinary complaints of incontinence.

- Urodynamic study shows the presence of hyper-reflexic type of bladder, which clearly indicates presence of cord dysfunction leading to neurogenic bladder, as compared to the hypertonic bladder seen in muscular disease.

*Neurological complaints*

- Lower extremity weakness
- Alterations in deep tendon reflexes

*Neurocutaneous markers of underlying spinal dysraphism*

- Nevus
- Hairy

*Musculoskeletal signs*

- Club foot and other foot deformities

## Suggested Readings

Bao N, Chen ZH, Gu S, Chen QM, Jin HM, Shi CR. Tight filum terminal syndrome in children: Analysis based on positioning of the conus and absence or presence of lumbosacral lipoma. *Child's Nerv Syst* 2007; **23**(10):1129–1134.

Di X. Endoscopic spinal tethered cord release: Operative technique. *Child's Nerv Syst* 2009; **25**(5):577–581.

Selçuki M, Coşkun K. Management of tight filum terminal syndrome with special emphasis on normal level conus medullaris (NLCM). *Surg Neurol* 1998; **50**(4):318–322; discussion 322.

Selden NR, Nixon RR, Skoog SR, Lashley DB. Minimal tethered cord syndrome associated with thickening of the terminal filum. *J Neurosurg* 2006; **105**(3 Suppl):214–218.

## Chapter 18

# Tethered Cord Syndrome

## Definition

Tethered cord syndrome (TCS) is a stretch-induced functional disorder of the spinal cord, resulting from excessive tension or traction that develops between two relatively fixed points, namely the lowest pair of attachment of the dentate ligament corresponding to spinal level T12–L1 and the conus medullaris anchored by inelastic structures. As a result of this fixation, the cord is prevented from its natural ascent during the first few months of life. This condition subsequently results in progressive neurological deficits secondary to traction of the conus medullaris.

Ischemia and hypoxia of the distal spinal cord, i.e. the conus has been implicated as the underlying pathophysiology of tethered cord syndrome. Common presenting complaints include neuro-orthopedic and urological deficits which are progressive in nature.

## Historical Perspective

The very first description of this clinical entity was made in 1910 by a physician named Fuchs who observed the association between severe degrees of spinal flexion and worsening of bladder continence in children with MMCL. He assumed that the increasing tension or traction on the distal spinal cord was responsible for this deterioration. In 1953, another physician named Garceau coined the term "filum terminal syndrome" for this unusual occurrence and concluded that a tight and inelastic filum terminal was accountable for the increased tension in the conus and subsequent neurological dysfunction. Finally in 1976, Hoffman et al. presented the first surgical series on untethering of cord and also discussed the improved clinical condition of cases that underwent untethering procedure.

## Embryology

The embryology of the human central nervous system involves two distinct stages: primary neurulation, followed by secondary neurulation process. The entire process starts during stage 8 of embryonic life and terminates at stage 14, corresponding to approximately days 18 to 32 of intrauterine development. The details of this embryological process have been described in previous sections.

Primary neurulation is a complex process during which the entire central nervous system is developed. However, the spinal cord segments pertaining to the sacral and the coccygeal segments develop during the secondary neurulation process. Primary neurulation occurs during embryonic stages 8 to 20 (days 18–48) and in the remaining period from 48 days onwards the secondary neurulation process takes place. Some of the conditions responsible for TCS are discussed below.

## Lipomyelomeningocele

Spinal lipoma or lipomyelomeningocele is the most common cause of primary tethered cord syndrome. It usually presents in infancy with a very conspicuous subcutaneous mass in the lower lumbar or sacral area. A radiological imaging undertaken by a diligent pediatrician reveals this occult spinal dysraphic state. The pathology involved in this spinal dysraphic state with lumbosacral lipoma is that the neural placode is outside the spinal canal and is intermingled with subcutaneous fatty tissue/through the defect in the vertebral lamina which tethers the conus medullaris.

## Thick filum terminale

The presence of fatty or fibrofatty tissue in the filum terminale leads to a diagnosis of tethered cord syndrome. The diagnosis is based on radiological imaging with MRI, correlating with clinical picture of terminal cord dysfunction like urological complaints.

## Terminal myelocystocele

The persistence of the fifth ventricle with tethering of the cord is a rare cause of tethered cord syndrome.

## Secondary Tethered Cord Syndrome

The occurrence of late onset neurological deterioration in children with previous repair of myelomeningocele should prompt the treating physician to perform an MRI imaging for evaluation of spinal cord tethering. The following are conditions most commonly seen with secondary tethered cord syndrome:

- Myelomeningocele
- Diastematomyelia
- Meningocele
- Dermal sinus
- Intradural spinal; tumors such as dermoid/epidermoid tumors

## Criteria for Diagnosis of Tethered Cord Syndrome

The diagnosis of tethered cord syndrome is one of combined radiological finding in conjunction with clinical correlation.

### Radiological criteria include an MRI picture, described as follows:

- Conus below vertebral body of L2
- Diameter of filum terminal >2 mm

Tethered cord syndrome has been classically described with low lying conus. However, there are variations present at the terminal end of the spinal cord. To add to the confusion, cases with normal level of conus may demonstrate symptoms compatible with TCS and the condition has been rightly named *occult tethered cord syndrome*. Therefore the primary question put forth is: What is the normal range of termination of the conus medullaris? In their autopsy studies, Reimann and Anson found that the cord ends at or above the inferior aspect of L2 vertebral body in 95% of the normal adult population but in 57% of the normal adult population the cord ends at or above the disc space of L1–L2. Thus the conclusion was that TCS can occur even with a normal position of the conus. Usually the cord achieves its adult position approximately by three months of postnatal life in a full term pregnancy.

Mechanical causes of cord tethering include thickening of filum terminal or one of the causes mentioned below:

- Fibrous or fibroadipose thickening of the filum
- Lumbosacral lipoma or lipomyelomeningocele
- Osseous or dural septum in diastematomyelia
- Scarring

These abovementioned structures lack elasticity and thus result in abnormal fixation of the cord.

## Pathogenesis of Tethered Cord Syndrome

The various theories regarding tethered cord syndrome are discussed here in detail with conclusion drawn from animal model experiments. Much of our understanding of the pathophysiology of TCS comes from animal model experiments and retrospective data on clinical features reported in the literature. Among the animal model experiments, the most useful evidence comes from feline model of TCS.

The experiment performed by Yamada *et al.* involved applying traction forces to the terminal part of the animal's spinal cord using various weights and then noting any neurophysiologic and metabolic changes in the spinal cord.

### Conclusion from the animal model experiments

The conclusion drawn from the abovementioned animal experiments were similar:

Any form of traction injury to the conus medullaris, i.e. the distal segment of the spinal cord, results in clinical symptoms which are compatible with either ischemic or metabolic dysfunction, or both.

It is evident that tethered cord syndrome is a traction-induced neuro-physiological disorder. The clinical features of TCS are explained here.

## Explaining TCS at the Neuroanatomical Level

The most common clinical presentation of TCS is sensorimotor complaints of lower limbs followed by urological issues and lastly by orthopedic and pain complaints, seen in pediatric onset of TCS. The spinal cord segment affected in TCS is localized at the lumbar or lumbosacral segment with subsequent involvement of the lumbosacral plexus, thus raising the question: Why is the lumbosacral segment of the cord most vulnerable to spinal cord tethering? This can be explained as follows: The lumbosacral plexus is the main nerve supply to the lower limb through the Onuf's nucleus, which is the lower motor control of micturition, also called the spinal urinary control center in the sacral segments S2, S3 and S4.

In the human spinal cord, there is presence of thick collagen bundles called *denticulate ligaments* that attach the dura laterally and then merge with the subpia medially. These denticulate ligaments are thought to provide stability to the spinal cord and they terminate at lower thoracic segment of T12 to L1.

From experimental studies, it has been shown that when the cord is stretched vertically, the elongation is greatest at the lower segments as compared to the upper segments. Hence it can be inferred that the most common site for neuronal dysfunction in TCS is the lumbosacral segment, i.e. below T12–L1, which lies below the lowest attachment of the dentate ligament.

Dysfunction of axons or nerve roots with their nuclei in spinal gray matter is called lower motor neuron (LMN) lesion. LMN lesions are not always caused by stretching of the cord but can arise from compression of nerve root or cord by a mass such as lipoma. Local dysgenesis of lower motor neurons, arising as a continuum of the original pathological process of spine bifida can also result in LMN dysfunction. Early signs of LMN lesion include orthopedic issues such as asymmetric development of lower limbs or club foot due to neuromuscular imbalance.

Presence of any neurological dysfunction of long fiber tracts originating from the brain such as spasticity of the legs should alert the treating physician to think of concurrent pathology such as presence of a syrinx in the upper cord. This possibility should be evaluated by ordering an MRI imaging of the whole spine.

## Vascular compromise

It has been noted that when traction forces are applied to the spinal cord, the blood vessels supplying the cord are stretched and constricted subsequently. The main point of constriction of blood vessels occurrs between the L2 and L3 segments. This segment corresponds to a watershed area, meaning there is poor collateral flow (the radicular artery of Adamkiewicz supplies the lumbosacral cord).

Thus it can be safely concluded that the lumbosacral segment is more vulnerable to ischemia than other cord segments.

Denticulate ligaments prevent rostral extension of the tension, or the traction force generated due to tethering of the distal cord. Vasogenic compromise or ischemia is one of the possible mechanisms underlying pathophysiology of TCS causing long nerve tract dysfunction.

## Neurophysiological basis of symptoms in TCS

From spinal cord injury models it is well known that the gray motor neuron depends heavily on oxidative metabolism for its functional integrity. In other words, they probably require more oxygen than white matter fibers do. This indicates the vulnerability of the gray matter neurons to ischemia of even mild degrees. The gray matter is where the anterior horn cells, interneuron and synaptic terminals of long descending tracts like corticospinal tract, are present.

### Short-latency somatosensory evoked potential (SSEP)

SSEP changes in the cord are concurrent with metabolic changes seen when traction forces are applied to the cord. This test shows the integrity of the sensory pathways and helps localization of conduction defects. After stimulation of a peripheral nerve, the impulses are recorded from the lower lumbar spinal cord/cervical cord and the sensory motor cortex.

For the lower limbs, either the peroneal nerve from the knee or the tibial nerve from the ankle is used. Somatosensory evoked potential changes are sensitive indicators of neurophysiological dysfunction. The following are changes seen in the cat's spinal cord by applying various degrees of traction forces:

Loss of all long tract potentials was observed during periods of traction and this was correlated with the metabolic changes indicative of hypoxia. The changes were reversible only with mild to moderate degree of traction similar to the metabolic changes.

From histopathological sections of animal studies, the presence of neuronal membrane wrinkling indicative of hypoxia was noted.

From the observations made by Yamada *et al.*, it was concluded that alterations in oxidative metabolism occurs in TCS in a similar pattern as it would occur in brain and spinal cord during periods of ischemia or hypoxia. Due to its extreme sensitivity to ischemia, it is gray matter dysfunction that leads to clinical symptoms in TCS.

## Biochemical basis of TCS

*Oxidative metabolic changes and redox ratio*

Redox ratio is the oxidation/reduction ratio of oxidative metabolism taking place in electron transport chain in the mitochondria. In other words, redox ratio is an indicator of adequate oxygen supply to the tissues with equally adequate blood supply. The reduction in the redox ratio is indicative of better oxygenation. As we have seen from the animal model experiments, there were definitive shifts in this redox ratio with onset of cord traction and ended with removal of the traction forces. This finding coincided with reversal of neurological dysfunction. Another method of showing hypoxic ischemia is the measurement of SSEP, which showed complete loss of electric potentials during period of hypoxic ischemia with reversal of these changes upon removal of traction forces. The oxidation/reduction ratio was measured in human lumbosacral cord during the procedure of untethering using a reflection spectrophotometer, a non-invasive method. The results of this investigation showed the reversibility of the redox potential changes after the untethering procedure. Schneider *et al.* performed color Doppler study during the untethering procedure and reported restoration of blood flow after untethering of cord.

## Conclusion

There is a definite change in the neuronal function seen in tethered cord syndrome. What is yet to be known is whether these dysfunctions result from mechanical stretch injury or ischemic compromise.

## Clinical Presentations

The clinical picture can be classified in the following categories:

i. Cutaneous
ii. Neurological-orthopedic

iii. Urological dysfunction

i. *Cutaneous markers*:

Presence of the following cutaneous signs should alert the pediatrician for radiological evaluation of the spine and to look for any sign of tethering of the conus. The cutaneous stigmata of occult spinal dysraphism are seen in >50% of children with TCS. The description of each of these cutaneous markers has been described elsewhere and only a brief revision is undertaken here as follows:

- Lumbosacral lipoma
- Lumbosacral hemangiomas
- Lumbosacral hypertrichosis (which is seen in 100% of diastemato-myelia cases)
- Dermal sinus
- Skin appendage

The presence of isolated capillary nevus (called nevus flammeus neonatorum) in the cervical region or isolated coccygeal dimple at the level of the gluteal fold has very weak association with occult spinal dysraphism.

ii. *Neuro-orthopedic symptoms*:

**Neurological symptoms**: In children, motor complaints dominate over sensory complaints and pain is hardly ever the presenting complaint. Contrary to children with TCS, in adults with TCS, pain is the most important presentation. Here the motor complaints are described along with their clinical explanation.

**Motor complaints**: In children, usual presentation include weakness of legs manifested as gait abnormality or dragging of foot. Complaints of being clumsy with frequent falls and tripping over are observed.

*Infants*: Observe for asymmetric movements or length of legs.

*Toddler*: Look for delayed walking ability or gait instability, or inquire about loss of previously acquired motor skills.

*Older children*: Inability to walk on heels or dragging of feet from weakness of ankle dorsiflexion. Muscle atrophy with hyporeflexia and hypotonia (sign of LMN lesion, local compression) is more common than UMN lesion (long tracts sign) of clonus and rigidity. Muscle atrophy is difficult to detect in infants due to presence of subcutaneous fat. Difference of more than 10% of muscle bulk at mid-thigh or calf

*Neural Tube Defects*

level is indicative of muscle atrophy. Spastic weakness of lower limbs
with hyper-reflexia (signs of UMN lesion).

   In the case of lumbosacral lipoma there may be asymmetrical motor
findings. The child in the image below has asymmetric feet and absence
of plantar creases, which may indicate impaired L5–S1 control.

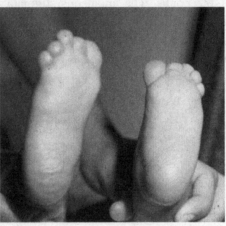

**Sensory complaints**: Pain as a presenting complaint is more common
in older children and adults. Non-dermatomal pattern of sensory
complaints like pain or paresthesias is mainly restricted to the feet
and perineum. In the case of paresthesias, the child usually describes
funny sensation of fuzzy feeling in the legs. Loss of pinprick sensation
is a common sensory finding.

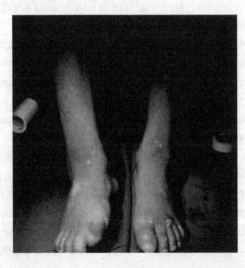

Rarely is there a complication from trophic ulcers (ulcer that develops from repeated injury arising from sensory deficits) as observed on the feet of this child from Mexico who had an untreated lumbosacral lipoma.

These sensory complaints may be masked in younger children because the symptoms can present as irritability and may be confused as night terrors or temper tantrums.

**Orthopedic complaints**: Orthopedic symptoms develop mostly due to the imbalance of nerve innervations and result in the following deformities:

- Cavovarus deformity, i.e. in-turned foot
- Cavovalgus deformity, i.e. foot rotated outward
- Club foot, i.e. equinovarus deformity of foot
- Scoliosis, i.e. curvature of spine
- Asymmetrical of limb lengths

**Club foot**: Since club foot is the most common orthopedic feature seen in children with spinal dysraphism and TCS, this clinical entity is described in detail here. Classic talipes equinovarus or club foot cases show the following three features:

- Equinus or plantar flexion of the leg at the ankle joint
- Varus or inversion deformity of the heel
- Forefoot adduction or in-turned foot

Any child with club foot deformity at birth should undergo examination of the spine (clinical and radiological exams like MRI) to rule out spinal dysraphism and also concurrent presence of any anorectal malformations.

**Scoliosis**: Scoliosis is another condition seen commonly in children with TCS.

*Definition*: Lateral curvature of the spine. Scoliosis is always associated with some rotation of the vertebrae.

*Most common location*: Thoracic spine.

*Examination*: Forward bending test. This test can detect early abnormalities of rotation that are not apparent when the patient is standing erect. The test is as follows: the child is asked to bend forward to a 90° angle with the hands joined in the middle and to look for any degree of rotation of the trunk or asymmetry of the paravertebral muscles.

*Diagnostic imaging*: X-ray spine in standing position. Presence of any left thoracic curvature should be considered with suspicion of underlying neurological condition like myelodysplasia.

*Treatment planning*:

- Curvatures <20° require no treatment.
- Curvatures between 20° and 40° will require bracing in skeletally immature child.
- Curvatures >60° are correlated with poor pulmonary functions and are candidates for spinal fusion surgeries.

iii. *Urological complaints*:
Urological issues warrant special description as it carries two important impacts: from the medical point of view to prevent renal complications, and from the social point of view to achieve proper continence. The following are types of urological manifestations seen:

- Overactive bladder manifests clinically as increased frequency/ urgency, nocturia or urge incontinence
- Increased frequency of urinary tract infections
- Urinary dribbling or involuntary urination
- Nocturnal enuresis
- Delayed toilet training

Sacral level of spina bifida is compatible with excellent mobility but the patient may suffer from severe bladder dysfunction.

## Role of videourodynamics

Neither clinical history of voiding habits nor normal neurological examination is reliable indicator of bladder dysfunction. Here comes the important role of videourodynamics as a sensitive test for early detection of bladder dysfunction, even before alteration in bladder status or evolution of any neurological deficit becomes evident.

**Urological assessment during the first three years of life in a child with TCS**

A child diagnosed with spinal dysraphism should undergo the following urological investigations:

- Urine analysis with periodic culture
- Renal function test — serum creatinine, serum electrolytes, blood urea nitrogen, ultrasound kidney, cystourethrography
- Urodynamic assessment

The last two tests, namely the urodynamic studies and the cystourethrography, are especially important in detecting early signs of cord damage.

The following are signs of UMN (upper motor neuron) dysfunction of bladder seen in cystourethrography:

- Small bladder with trabeculation due to uninhibited contractions of detrusor muscle of the bladder wall
- Vesicoureteral reflux indicative of high bladder pressure

The following are signs of LMN (lower motor neuron) dysfunction of bladder seen in cystourethrography:

- Large atonic bladder
- Open bladder neck

Serial videourodynamic studies are the gold standard for evaluating bladder dysfunction.

**Cystometrogram (CMG):** A graphic representation of bladder pressure as a function of filling volume. In cystometrogram, UMN dysfunction is detected by the presence of bladder hyperactivity (uninhibited bladder contractions) and incomplete bladder emptying.

**Electromyography (EMG):** EMG of external urethral sphincter during bladder filling and emptying is performed with dysnergic sphincter activity during bladder contractions, i.e. persistently low level of EMG activity or increased EMG spikes are signs of UMN dysfunction.

**Complications of bladder dysfunction in children with TCS**

Repeated cystitis with ascent of infection to upper urinary tract result in pyelonephritis and renal scarring. Detrusor sphincter dysnergia, a condition where there is dissociation between bladder contraction and receptive relaxation of the external urethral sphincter, is another possible complication. This leads to obstruction and incomplete voiding. Vesicoureteral reflux with possible progression to hydronephrosis and ultimately chronic renal dysfunction is ultimately the most dreaded complication.

**Differential diagnosis of urinary incontinence in children: Hinman syndrome**

Hinman syndrome or non-neurogenic bladder dysfunction is a condition seen in children with behavioral abnormality or developmental delay. Even the urodynamics testing may show a false positive presence of hyperactive bladder or detrusor sphincter dysnergia. However, this condition improves with age and training.

**TCS-associated syndromes**

These syndromes need to be evaluated from the neurosurgical point of view.

1. **Caudal agenesis**: Caudal regression syndrome/segmental dysgenesis syndrome
2. **Anorectal atresia syndromes**
   - **OEIS**: Omphalocele, exstrophy of bladder, imperforate anus, spina bifida
   - **VACTERL**: Vertebral anomaly, anus imperforate, tracheoesophageal fistula, radii abnormality
   - **Currarino's triad**: Autosomal dominant condition consisting of triad of bony sacral defect, anorectal malformation and presacral mass like a teratoma or anterior myelomeningocele, or a combination of both.

**Isolated anorectal anomalies seen in TCS**: About 10–50% of cases with occult spinal dysraphism will have an element of anorectal malformation. Common clinical conditions are:

- Cloacal exstrophy

- Imperforate anus
- Anal atresia
- Renal dysplasia
- Bladder exstrophy

## Diagnostic Investigations of TCS

**MRI**: The diagnostic imaging modality of choice in suspected cases of TCS is the MRI spine. T1 sagittal image is especially useful to detect fat in the filum. Associated anomalies can also be detected. The diagnostic power of MRI is very high in cases where the cord is distinctively below L3, whereas in cases where the cord ends between L1 and L2, the radiological criteria is also very helpful.

In children with MMCL the level of tethering corresponds to one of the original levels of defect, whereas in children with thickened filum terminale, the TCS level can range the whole length of the cauda equina.

### Ancillary tests

**CT with CT myelogram**: The CT myelogram is used only when MRI cannot be performed. This test is not very popular in children as it is invasive. However, the position of roots can be better identified using CT myelogram than MRI.

**X-ray spine**: Although x-ray spine is very useful to detect osseous anomalies like bifid vertebra or hemivertebrae, its usefulness is limited to delineation of scoliosis and orthopedic procedures.

**Vertebral anomalies**: Bony anomalies are seen in 95% of TCS cases and include the following:

- Bifid vertebrae
- Laminar defects
- Hemivertebrae
- Sacral aplasia/sacral agenesis
- Multiple segmentation error

Presence of bifid spinous process at L5–S1 level is seen in 30% of normal population of children aged between one and ten years.

## Surgery

As expressed in the chapter about surgical indication for lipomas, we realize that there are two different opinions. Either overstretching or pathological tension in the cord along with shortened nerve roots could be the reason why ascent of the conus is not seen after untethering of cord in most of the cases. Thus radiological imaging must always be correlated with the clinical picture.

### Clinical outcome after untethering of cord

Common clinical manifestations of tethered cord syndrome include neuro-orthopedic features combined with urological and pain complaints. In cases of scoliosis with curvature of less than 50°, cord untethering procedure improved or stabilized the curve in the majority of the cases (63%); however, improvement of the curve was less when the curvature was greater than 50°. Similar result has been observed for improvement of kyphosis after untethering procedure. From the neurological standpoint, children who underwent contracture release without untethering procedure continued to experience worsening of their contractures and required subsequent repeated contracture release procedures as compared to children whose condition stabilized after untethering of cord. The incidence cited in the literature is as high as 79% improvement in motor functions and close to 100% improvement in pain and other sensory complaints.

In the case of bladder complaints, frequent catheterization and worsening of urinary incontinence in a child with MMCL indicate underlying retethering of the cord. The most common urodynamic study shows areflexic detrusor dysfunction. An improvement in neurogenic bladder is seen in as high as 60% of cases after untethering of cord. In addition, for children who did not undergo cord untethering procedure and instead underwent contractures release, on long-term follow-up it was revealed that this group of children required bladder augmentation surgeries as they developed worsening of incontinence.

In conclusion, children with operated MMCL should be followed clinically for appearance of any deterioration of clinical symptoms to detect tethered cord syndrome at an early stage.

## Secondary tethered cord syndrome in MMCL children with repair of defect at birth

Tethered spinal cord occurs in 3–15% of cases with a history of repaired myelomeningocele. Symptomatic tethering may result from scarring or adhesive arachnoiditis involving the neural placode with secondary adherence of the cord to the overlying fascia or dura mater.

The clinical manifestations are in the form of clinical deterioration of pre-existing symptoms. However, the treating physician should rule out other causes masquerading as tethered cord syndrome such as shunt malfunction, Chiari malformation and syringomyelia. A routine MRI spine will help to delineate the specific underlying pathology.

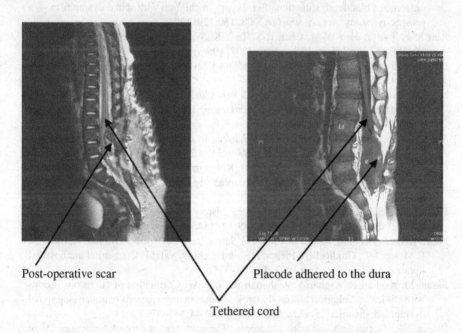

Post-operative scar                    Placode adhered to the dura

Tethered cord

The image on the left corresponds to a child who had surgery for resection of lumbosacral lipoma while the image on the right corresponds to one who had myelomeningocele repair.

The persistence of tethering after surgery, as demonstrated in the figure, brings to mind the debate about the surgical indications for lipomas. The issue has been discussed in the corresponding chapter.

## Suggested Readings

Bademci G, Saygun M, Batay F, *et al.* Prevalence of primary tethered cord syndrome associated with occult spinal dysraphism in primary school children in Turkey. *Pediatr Neurosurg* 2006; **42**:4–13.

Bui CJ, Tubbs RS, Oakes J. Tethered cord syndrome in children: A review. *Neurosurg Focus* 2007; **23**(2):E2.

Daryl E. Warder. Tethered cord syndrome and occult spinal dysraphism. *Neurosurg Focus* 2001; 15;**10**(1):E1.

Drake J. Occult tethered cord syndrome: Not an indication for surgery. *J Neurosurg* 2006; **104**(5):305–308.

Koyanagi I, Yoshinobu I, Hida K, Abe H, Isu T, Akino M. Surgical treatment supposed natural history of the tethered cord with occult spinal dysraphism. *Child's Nerv Syst* 1997; **13**:268–274.

Kumar R, Singhal N, Gupta M, Kapoor R, Mahapatra AK. Evaluation of clinico-urodynamic outcome of bladder dysfunction after surgery in children with spinal dysraphism — a prospective study. *Acta Neurochir* 2008; **150**:129–137.

Kuo M-F, Tsai Y, Hsu W-M, Chen R-S, Tu Y-K, Wang H-S. Tethered spinal cord and VACTERL association. *J Neurosurg* 2007; **106**(3):201–204.

Lew SM, Kothbauer KF. Tethered cord syndrome: An updated review. *Pediatr Neurosurg* 2007; **43**:236–248.

Macejko AM, Cheng EY, Yerkes EB, Meyer T, Bowman RM, Kaplan WE. Clinical urological outcomes following primary tethered cord release in children younger than three years. *J Urol* 2007; **178**:1738–1743.

Michelson D, Ashwal S. Tethered cord syndrome in childhood: Diagnostic features and relationship to congenital anomalies. *Neurol Res* 2004; **26**(7):745–753.

Ohe N, Futamura A, Kawada R, Minatsu H, Kohmura H, Hayashi K, Miwa K, Sakai N. Secondary tethered cord syndrome in spinal dysraphism. *Child's Nerv Syst* 2000; **16**:457–461.

Phuong LK, Schoeberl K, Raffel C. Natural history of tethered cord in patients with meningomyelocele. *Neurosurg* 2002; **89**(12):1545–1550.

Pierre-Kahn A, Zerah M, Renier D, Cinalli G, Sainte-Rose C, Lellouch-Tubiana A, Brunelle F, Merrer ML, Giudicelli Y, Pichon J, Kleinknecht B, Nataf F. Congenital lumbosacral lipomas. *Child's Nerv Syst* 1997; **13**:298–335.

Sasani M, Asghari B, Asghari Y, Afsharian R, Ozer AF. Correlation of cutaneous lesions with clinical radiological and urodynamic findings in the prognosis of underlying spinal dysraphism disorders. *Pediatr Neurosurg* 2008; **44**:360–370.

Selden NR. Occult tethered cord syndrome: The case for surgery. *J Neurosurg* 2006; **104**:302–304.

Steinbok P, Garton G, Gupta N. Occult tethered cord syndrome: A survey of practice patterns. *J Neurosurg* 2006; **104**(5):309–313.

Tarcan T, Önol FF, lker YI, Imek FS, Özek M. Does surgical release of secondary spinal cord tethering improve the prognosis of neurogenic bladder in children with myelomeningocele. *J Urol* 2006; **176**:1601–1606.

Yamada S, Knerium DS, Mandybur GM, Schultz RL and Yamada BS. Pathophysiology of tethered cord syndrome and other complex factors. *Neurol Res* 2004; **26**(7):722–726.

Yamada S, Won DJ, Yamada SM. Pathophysiology of tethered cord syndrome: Correlation with symptomatology. *Neurosurg Focus* 2004; 15;**16**(2):E6.

# Chapter 19

# Syringomyelia

## Definition

Syringomyelia is derived from the Greek word *syrinx*, meaning "pipe" or "tube". Syringomyelia is a disorder in which the central cavitations within the spinal cord lead to progressive degeneration of the spinal cord. The classic clinical picture of syringomyelia is brachial amyotrophy, which present as painless burns, subsequently result in weakness and wasting of the small muscles in the hand.

This disorder is commonly but not obligatorily associated with NTD. Below we will expand on the general characteristics of syringomyelia even if they are not directly related to patients with NTD. Certainly many of the symptoms that will be described below vary in its presentations according to the clinical condition of the child. In high lesion MMCL, the warning signs of an impinging syrinx will be different from a child with a lower lesion. Nonetheless, the symptoms secondary to a cervical syringomyelia or syringobulbia will be the same in almost every patient with associated NTD.

## Historical Perspective

The earliest description of syringomyelia can be dated back to the 16th century when the French anatomist, Etienne Geoffroy Saint-Hilaire mentioned the presence of a cavity within the spinal cord in his monograph *La Dissection du Corps Human*. This was followed by Giovanni Battista Morgagni in 1740, who recognized the cystic nature of the condition. However, it was Olivier d'Angers in 1827 who coined the term syringomyelia. Throughout the history of medicine, there has been confusion regarding the true pathophysiology of syringomyelia. In the 19th century, hydromyelia was the new term introduced replacing syringomyelia. In 1943, Ingraham and Scott noted spinal cord cavitations in autopsy specimens of children with myelomeningocele. The association between syringomyelia and myelomeningocele was further strengthened by Cameron *et al.* in necropsy series of children with myelomeningocele. Cameron reported an incidence of 77% and also noticed that many of these children had severe internal hydrocephalus. This feature led many physicians to believe that syringomyelia was an aftermath of hydrocephalus. Although true, syringomyelia can also arise from other etiopathologies and this will be discussed in detail in the following section.

In this text, differentiation between syringomyelia and hydromyelia are made with syringomyelia being used in the context of spinal cord cavitations and hydromyelia reserved for dilations of central canal.

## Incidence and Prevalence of Syrinx

Here we describe syringomyelia only in association with spina bifida. The true incidence of this clinical entity is underestimated as many cases remain asymptomatic. In addition, before the advent of MRI, the diagnoses of syringes were made mainly based on clinical presentations or as an autopsy finding.

MRI of syringes with incidence of 20–53% in open spinal dysraphism is noted. From the literature, the incidence of syringomyelia detected in autopsy of children with myelomeningocele was reported with an incidence that ranged from 42% to 77%. Many of these children had died as a complication of severe internal hydrocephalus and this led the then treating physicians to believe syringomyelia to be a direct effect of hydrocephalus.

The reported incidence of syringomyelia with diastematomyelia is 29–35%. With spinal lipoma the incidence is around 11–27% with equal distribution between lipomyelomeningocele and fatty filum terminale with an incidence of 20% for each. In a large study by Pierre-Kahn, the incidence of syringomyelia was noted to be 23%, however only 9.3% were found to be symptomatic. Furthermore, dilations of the central canal were excluded from this study.

### Site involved

The most common location of a syrinx is the cervical spine. It usually involves segments C8 to T1. Upward extension of the cavity into the lower brain stem is called *syringobulbia*, which can present with lower cranial nerve dysfunction. The following images show MRI spine of a child with L4 myelomeningocele.

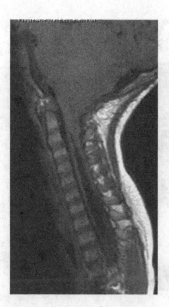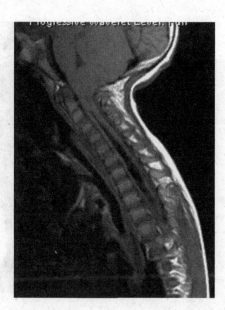

Syrinx in the lower cord is seen commonly in association with closed spinal dysraphism and accompanying tethered cord syndrome. But the image below belongs to the same child as the images above. His lesion extended almost the entirety of the cord. Eventually it was controlled by revising the shunt, in spite of the child not having any signs and symptoms of classical hydrocephalus.

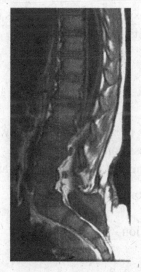

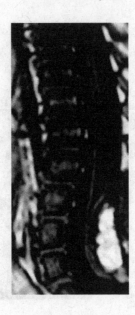

The above image belongs to a child with a lumbar lipoma. The syrinx was related to the tethered cord. The precise mechanism for this association is not well understood.

## Classification

The first classification of syringes is based on its origin while the second classification is based on its pathophysiology.

### Etiological classification

i. *Congenital causes*

1. **Chiari type I** is the most common etiology.
2. **Chiari type II** is less commonly involved.
3. **Craniocervical junction anomalies** such as

   - Klippel–Feil deformity
   - Platybasia
   - Basilar invagination

ii. *Acquired causes*

- Intramedullary tumor like astrocytoma or meningioma
- Traumatic syringomyelia
- Hemorrhagic necrosis of spinal cord

## Modified Barnett classification

**Type I**: Obstruction of foramen magnum with dilatation of the central canal, associated with Chiari type I and other obstructive lesions at the foramen magnum.

**Type II**: Syringomyelia without obstruction at the foramen magnum.

**Type III**: Acquired disease of the spinal cord.

- Spinal cord tumors (usually intramedullary tumors)
- Traumatic myelopathy
- Spinal arachnoiditis with pachymeningitis
- Secondary myelomalacia from cord compression (tumor/trauma), infarction, hematomyelia

## Origin of Syringomyelia

### Classical theories of formation of syrinx

Both Gardner and Williams hypothesized the formation of syringomyelia based on the concept that transmission of CSF from the fourth ventricle to the syrinx cavity occurs via a patent central canal.

### Gardner's hydrodynamic theory of formation of syrinx

According to Gardner, the fluid in the syrinx originate from the supratentorial CSF. He hypothesized that obstruction to the outflow of CSF via the foramen of Magendie or block at the foramen magnum resulted in a secondary generation of augmented ventricular pressure pulses. Thus these increased positive pressure pulses act like a water hammer and transfer the forces to the spinal canal via the CSF fluid, leading to formation of a syrinx.

## Williams' craniospinal dissociation theory

According to this theory, during valsalva maneuvers there is a block created by the cerebellar tonsils at the foramen magnum, which acts like a one-way valve to prevent the rise of intracranial pressure. Thus a pressure gradient is created between the spinal CSF spaces and intracranial CSF spaces. With any degree of herniation of the cerebellar tonsils as seen in Chiari malformations, there is a block created at the level of foramen magnum, which exacerbates this craniospinal pressure dissociation. This results in low spinal pressure and high intracranial pressure. Thus a sucking effect is created, which draws fluid into the low-pressure spinal canal and results in the development of syringomyelia.

These abovementioned theories could not explain the syringes at more caudal location of the cord. Moreover, if the syrinx is formed due to a foramen magnum block, then the severity of the syrinx should correlate with higher locations in the cord according to severity of the block.

## Piston theory of formation of syringomyelia

Oldfield *et al.* proposed the Piston Theory of syringomyelia and this theory has been considered relevant to the origin of syringomyelia since then. According to them, the herniation or increased downward movement of the cerebellar tonsil acts like a piston on the partly obstructed spinal subarachnoid space at the level of foramen magnum. With the physiological increase in CSF pressure during cardiac systole, the cranial part of the subarachnoid CSF is compressed and forced through the central canal, leading to expansion of the distal part of the syrinx cavity. This hypothesis is similar to Williams' hypothesis of presence of suction effect and he named it the "slosh phenomenon".

## Pathophysiology of Syringomyelia

Based on radiological imaging and anatomical corelation, the symptoms of syringomyelia can be explained as follows. For purpose of explanation the syringes are divided into the following categories. These categories have been originally described based on axial MRI and are correlated with histopathological examination:

- Dilation of central canal
- Dilation of central canal with paracentral extension
- Eccentric dilation of spinal cord

## *Dilation of central canal*

This variant of syringomyelia is described as tubular dilations of central canal that is anatomically continuous with the fourth ventricle and is also referred to as "communicating syringomyelia" in the literature. It is seen in children more often than adults, with an average age of presentation of six years. It is most commonly seen with myelomeningocele and described in association with any conditions which interfere with CSF dynamics, such as Chiari malformation, Dandy–Walker syndrome, and hydrocephalus — in other words, any factors that can cause foramen magnum block.

With obstruction to the flow of CSF through the aqueduct and with development of adhesions to the outlet foramina of the fourth-ventricle, the fourth ventricle becomes isolated from the lateral ventricles with subsequent development of two compartments. Further aggravation to this situation is brought about by foramen magnum block to CSF pathway, such as herniation of cerebellar tonsils in Chiari malformation. The herniated tonsils compress the upper part of the syrinx and thus the syrinx assumes the typical configuration of having a larger diameter at its terminal segment.

## Pathological finding

From histopathological studies, such syringes have been noted to be lined with ependymal cells either completely or at times partially. Thus these syringes could possibly represent simple dilations of the central canal. With gross dilations of the central canal, the ependymal linings have been demonstrated only at the poles of the syrinx with most of them being covered by compressed glial tissue.

## Neurophysiology

From histopathological studies of syringes with dilation of central canal, the absence of neuronal cell death indicates that the symptoms seen with this variant of syrinx or hydromyelia are the result of compressive nervous dysfunction rather than cell necrosis. This means that there is stretching of long tracts without significant Wallerian degeneration. This might have an implication on the relatively better prognosis for recovery from neurological deficits seen in such patients.

## Clinical picture

Most patients are asymptomatic or pauci-symptomatic. When symptomatic, the neurological deficit conforms with central cord syndrome, i.e. with bilateral neurological deficits in the form of dissociative anesthesia, accompanied by weakness of the hands. Dissociative anesthesia is explained as loss of pain and temperature sensation with preservation of fine tactile and kinesthetic sensations (pressure, vibration and joint position senses). This is considered to be the classical picture of syringomyelia, and is also known as *brachial amyotrophy*.

## Explaining this classical picture from anatomical correlation

The central canal is surrounded by lamina X, which is the central gray matter. Right in front of lamina X are the decussating fibers of lateral spinothalamic tracts which carry pain and temperature sensations from the contralateral side of the body. These fibers are most affected by dilations of the central canal. On the other hand, the fibers carrying the tactile and kinesthetic sensations are located dorsally ascending ipsilaterally in the dorsal funiculus which are preferentially spared. The extension of the dilations towards the anterior or ventral horn of the spinal gray matter leads to segmental or lower motor neuron dysfunction which manifests as weakness of small muscles of hand, supplied by the ulnar nerve.

Thus the clinical picture brought about by dilation of the central canal can be explained bearing in mind this anatomical and neurophysiologic dysfunction. This type of syrinx is often mentioned in the literature as hydromyelia and it may be detected as an incidental finding in an asymptomatic or may be pauci-symptomatic patient. This finding is especially intriguing due to the large size and length of the syrinx. A significant correlation has been found with length of the syrinx and age of the patient, with larger syringes present in children with an average age of two years than in older children or young adults with age of 14 years and above. This phenomenon could be explained by age-related stenosis of the central canal.

### Central cavities with paracentral extensions and eccentric cavities

These two variants are grouped together as they share a similarity in terms of clinical presentation and prognosis.

The central cavities with paracentral extension could possibly represent dilations of the central canal with rupture of the syrinx at its weakest spots like its two poles. Needless to say, central cavity with paracentral extensions also arises from abnormal CSF dynamics. On the other hand, eccentric cavities represent cavitary lesions that develop as an aftermath of myelomalacia, rightly seen in conditions associated with spinal cord injury, which can be in the form of traumatic or ischemic injury.

### Clinical Presentations

Both these variants of syringomyelia are always symptomatic especially the eccentric cavities. The most common location of either paracentric or eccentric cavities is the posterolateral site. Thus the clinical picture is dominated by segmental clinical signs, which can be correlated well with the localization of the cavity by radiological imaging, in terms of spinal level of lesion, side of lesion and even the quadrant of lesion affected. The segmental clinical signs are dominated by sensory symptoms as explained above, the posterolateral preferential affection of the cord by the cavitary process. This locale of the cavitations or syrinx formation coincides with the watershed area with the possibility of an ischemic etiology of syringomyelia. The following are the types of clinical presentations:

- Spastic weakness of legs
- Segmental sensory loss
- Segmental presence of paresthesias and dysesthesia
- Upper extremity weakness

Atrophy is rarely seen due to involvement of the anterior horn cell from the anterolateral extension of the syrinx cavity. In children with myelomeningocele, the following complaints always warrant a diagnostic imaging in the form of MRI of brain and also of the whole spine:

- Lower back pain with occasional radicular type of pain.
- **Quality of pain**: Burning, aching and continuous.
- **Distribution**: Usually bilateral but unilateral sensory dysfunction has also been reported. This holds true for amyotrophy as well.
- **Location**: The sensory loss is distributed in a cape or hemicape pattern with extension to the back of head and trunk.
- **Modality of sensory loss**: The most commonly detected finding in sensory system examination in children with syringomyelia is the presence of dissociate loss of pain and temperature sensation with preservation of tactile, vibration and kinesthetic sensation. If the tactile sensation in the arms and hands are lost then there will be loss of vibration and position sense concomitantly. However, in the case of lower limbs, the situation is slightly different. There is usually some loss of pain and thermal sensation proximally and over the abdomen but more often there is loss of kinesthetic sensations in posterior columns, which forms the basis of sensory ataxia in lower limbs.

### Sensory examination

**Distribution**: Positive findings include loss of pain and temperature sensation in a cape-like distribution. There is relative sparing of tactile, vibration and position sensation with preservation of two-point discrimination as well.

**Location**: Involved areas include arms and hands and on the posterior side there is sensory dysfunction affecting the back of the neck, shoulders and slightly descending to the back.

**Spinal level**: Level of sensory dysfunction corresponds to C8 to T1 spinal segments.

**Associated findings**: Often patient present with painless ulcer on the hand secondary to insensitivity to pain or thermal stimuli. This ulcer which develops secondary to sensory nerve dysfunction is called a *trophic ulcer*. Due to repeated trauma secondary to insensitivity to pain and temperature sensations there are evidence of scarring and edema. Repeated trauma to small joints of the hand or the wrist may manifest as neuropathic joint, a clinical condition called *Charcot's joint*. In extreme cases with repeated trauma to fingers, autoamputation of terminal phalanges has been reported in the literature.

## Motor examination findings

Atrophy or reduction of the thenar and hypothenar eminences with difficulty in fine motor movements of the hand, especially worsening of handwriting and clumsiness, are common motor examination findings. Fasciculation, which are described as involuntary contractions of arm muscle group can be detected or demonstrated on EMG as fibrillations (only detected on EMG and are not visible clinically). This is a pathognomonic sign of lower motor neuron lesion. Finally, with extensive cavitations within the cord, syringomyelia then presents with spastic weakness and ataxia of the lower limbs (possibly from involvement of the decussating corticospinal tract), indicative of UMN dysfunction. Long cavities of syringomyelia can lead to appearance of lower motor neuron signs in all four extremities. With concomitant presence of Chiari, shoulders may be atrophic and hands spastic.

## Torticollis

Tonic deviation of the neck to one side is called *torticollis*. Appearance of torticollis may be an initial manifestation of cervical cavitations from injury to nerve roots of the spinal accessory nerve (cranial nerve number XI) which supplies the sternoclediomastoid muscle. Though rare, Chiari type II can also present clinically as torticollis.

## Bladder complaints

Due to interruption of the descending corticospinal tracts which carry information from the higher centers to the sacral micturition center called the Onuf's nucleus, the result is spastic bladder with involuntary voiding and increasing sense of urgency and frequency. This type of bladder with detrusor hypertonia is called *automatic bladder*.

## Orthopedic features

Kyphoscoliosis can also present in the setting of syringomyelia. The pathogenesis behind the development to scoliosis is weakness of paravertebral muscles.

**Autonomic disturbance**

The descending sympathetic fibers terminate at the stellate ganglion. The postganglionic fibers are distributed through C8 to T1 roots. Hence cervical syrinx cases might develop Horner's syndrome. The syndrome has the following constellation of signs from interruption of the sympathetic supply:

- *Miosis*: Constricted pupil from loss of sympathetic flow to constrictor pupillae muscle.
- *Ptosis*: Drooping of eyelids from loss of innervations to the levator palpebrae superioris.
- *Anhydrosis*: Lack of sweating of face and upper limbs from loss of innervations to the sweat glands.
- *Loss of ciliospinal reflex*: Applying painful stimuli to the nape of neck causes papillary constriction. This reflex is lost in Horner's syndrome.
- *Lower limb complaints*: Spastic weakness of legs manifests as dragging of feet or limping and gait instability. Inability to walk on toes (S1 spinal level) or inability to walk on heels (L5 spinal level) can localize the spinal segment. Sensory complaints are similar to upper extremity complaints, which have been described earlier, with paresthesias and dysesthesia. Case reports of sciatica-like pain has also been reported.

## Differential Diagnosis

### Conditions which masquerade as syringomyelia

The following conditions can have similar clinical picture as seen in syringomyelia. The pathologies described here are pertaining only to those conditions which are seen in spinal dysraphism (myelomeningocele):

*Upper extremity complaints*

- Chiari type II
- Posterior fossa or cervical arachnoid cyst
- Split cord malformation at cervical level
- Craniovertebral junction anomalies

*Lower extremity complaints*

- Tethered cord syndrome, either primary or secondary (retethering of cord seen after myelomeningocele repair). Most common occult spinal dysraphisms associated with syrinx are spinal lipomas and diastematomyelia.
- Intrinsic myelodysplasia as in myelomeningocele.

## Treatment

As syringomyelia is a condition of uncertain etiology and unpredictable evolution, it is not surprising that there are many surgical approaches to treat it.

As in any other pathology we have to be certain that the patient displays symptoms and that there is evidence of progression of the syrinx. It is important to obtain the opinion of a neuroradiologist who will differentiate a true syringomyelia from an enlarged or dilated central canal, the latter being a normal condition.

Specifically in cases of NTD we aim to determine if there is tethered cord; if so, then untether it.

In children with MMCL it is tempting to correlate their Chiari II with what we know about Chiari I and syringomyelia, conditions in which there is indeed an association between them, thus the treatment of the former controls the latter. But, as mentioned in the chapter about MMCL, the foramen magnum is enlarged and the cerebellar tonsils are adhered to the brain stem in such a way that exploring the foramens of Luschka and Magendie can cause severe harm to the child. So, in our opinion, the best approach is to revise the VP shunt or place one. The rationale for the revision is that the bulk of the CSF that enlarges the syrinx is produced in the lateral ventricles and optimizing the drainage of the CSF from there will reduce the fluid available for enlarging the syrinx. This is reasonable even if the ventricles seem to be unchanged. We have to factor in that the enlarging syrinx serves as a fifth ventricle.

There are surgeons who shunt the syrinx to the spinal arachnoid space or to the pleura. Personally I do not favor this approach but I do respect those who opt for this alternative. There are occasions in which it seems that nothing we do for the patient is working and provided there is a rationale behind, all alternatives should be brought forward and considered.

## Suggested Readings

Beaumont A, Muszynski CA, Kaufman BA. Clinical significance of terminal syringomyelia in association with pediatric tethered cord syndrome. *Pediatr Neurosurg* 2007; **43**:216–221.

Chang H, Nakagawa H. Hypothesis on the pathophysiology of syringomyelia based on simulation of cerebrospinal fluid dynamics. *J Neurol Neurosurg Psychiatry* 2003; **74**:344–347.

Dan Greitz. Unraveling the riddle of syringomyelia. *Neurosurg Rev* 2006; **29**:251–264.

Isu T, Chono Y, Iwasaki Y, Koyanagi I, Akino M, Abe H, Abumi K. Scoliosis associated with syringomyelia presenting in children. *Child's Nerv Syst* 1992; **8**:97–100.

Klekamp J. The pathophysiology of syringomyelia — historical overview and current concept. *Acta Neurochir* 2002; **144**:649–664.

Levine D. The pathogenesis of syringomyelia associated with lesions at the foramen magnum: A critical review of existing theories and proposal of a new hypothesis. *J Neurol Sci* 2004; **220**:3–21.

Milhorat T. Classification of syringomyelia. *Neurosurg Focus* 2000; 15:**8**(3):E1.

Milhorat T, Capocelli A, Anzil LA, Kotzen R, Milhorat R. Pathological basis of spinal cord cavitations in syringomyelia: Analysis of 105 autopsy cases. *J Neurosurg* 1995; **82**:802–812.

Piatt JH Jr. Syringomyelia complicating myelomeningocele: Review of the evidence. *J Neurosurg* 2004; **100**(2):101–109.

Royo-Salvador MB, Solé-Llenas J, Doménech JM, Gonzalez-Adrio R. Results of the section of the filum terminale in 20 patients with syringomyelia, scoliosis and Chiari malformation. *Acta Neurochir* (*Wien*) 2005; **147**:515–523.

Yeom JS, Lee CK, Park KW, Lee JH, Lee DH, Wang KC, Chang BS. Scoliosis associated with syringomyelia: Analysis of MRI and curve progression. *Eur Spine J* 2007; **16**:1629–1635.

Part II

# Cranial Defects

Chapter 20

# Anencephaly

## Definition

The classical definition by Lemire describes the partial or complete absence of the cranial vault with absence of overlying tissues and malformation and destruction of rudimentary brain structures. Exencephaly represents an antenatal diagnosis where there is protrusion of brain tissue before its degeneration, which is considered a step prior to anencephaly. Anencephaly is one of those NTD which is incompatible with prolonged extrauterine life. In 1984, Baird and Sadovnick published a study of 181 live-born anencephalics and found that 42.5% lived longer than 24 hours and 14.9% survived more than three days.

Since the advent of prenatal ultrasonography, there has been a different pattern of survival rates due to easy detection and legalization of abortions.

## Historical Perspective

In 1826, the zoologist and teratologist Etienne Saint-Hilaire described an Egyptian mummy with anencephaly. Since then, many examples and classification of anencephaly has been quoted. In 1987, an anencephalic infant became a donor for heart transplant, which opened the avenue for potential donor resources and also the debate of ethical issue as to when to declare an anencephalic infant brain dead.

## Incidence and Prevalence

- Incidence: 1 to 2 per 1000 live births
- Female preponderance is noted with incidence of 3:1 to 7:1
- The highest incidence in the world is in Western UK, with 3.17 to 10 per 1000 live births (1975)

## Molecular Genetics

- Most cases have normal chromosomal makeup.
- Anencephaly has also been reported in the following anomalies:

  1. Trisomy 18
  2. Trisomy 20
  3. Partial deletion of chromosome 13
  4. Duplication of chromosome 2

- There has been no consistent pattern of chromosomal pattern detected so far.

## Classification

Two types of anencephaly are seen:

- *Microacrania* (Microanencephaly): Occipital foramen is patent with normal foramen magnum.
- *Holocrania* (Holoanencephaly): Absence of great occipital foramen with extension into foramen magnum.

## Embryology

Muller and O'Rahilly in 1984 reported that anencephaly was determined at stage 8 (18 days after fertilization). According to them, the early development of the skull and brain occur independently and the brain of an anencephalic embryo differentiates before it degenerates and the cranial vault disturbance occurs before the brain degenerates.

There are three stages in formation of an anencephalic defect:

- Cerebral dysraphia beginning at stage 11.
- Exposure of the epencephalic brain throughout the later part of embryonic life.
- Degeneration of the exposed brain by the amniotic fluid and mechanical damage.

- Marin-Padilla's study showed that primary defects in the pathogenesis of all neural tube defects is due to mesodermal insufficiency.

Mesenchymal defect results in failure of the neural tube to elevate and failure of closure. Defect in the sphenoid bone has been postulated as the primary defect in anencephaly.

## Pathological Features of the Anencephalic Infant

### Head

Striking appearance of a red, shiny membranous mass called *area cerebrovasculosa*, present at the base of the skull.

Microscopic examination of the mass reveals the presence of hemorrhagic vascular structure with variable amount of connective tissue and occasional appearance of glial tissue with small twists of neurons, ependymal and choroid plexus.

Usually there is no membrane covering the area cerebrovasculosa.

### Note

Presence of any membrane or wisp on the area vasculosa should be examined for any amniotic tissue as it would represent the "amniotic rupture sequence" rather than the anencephaly of multifactorial type.

- The junction of the normal skin and the mass is a thin, bluish gray, translucent rim which on histological sections demonstrates the presence of keratinizing, stratified squamous epithelium lacking the skin appendages.
- Remnants of cerebral hemisphere are seen.
- The amount of brain tissue present posteriorly correlates with the amount of occipital bone covering.
- Presence of brain stem or cerebellum depends on whether the anencephaly is of meroacrania or holoacrania with presence of rudimentary brain stem and cerebellum present in the former.
- Descending tract is always absent in the brain stem.
- Eyes are of normal size which on microscopic examination showed total absence of neurons of the ganglion cell layer with hypoplasia of optic nerve fiber layer.
- Photoreceptor layer in the eye is complete and the inner nuclear layer is normal.

## Spine

- Spinal cord is present where the bony parts are covered with normal ventral horn cells and large central canal.
- Spinal column may be closed partially or open completely.
- Various vertebral anomalies may be present, especially retroflexion of the cervical spine.

## Bony Abnormalities

### Craniofacial abnormalities

- Triangular shape of skull.
- Small, narrow, short and anteriorly rotated sphenoid bone with prominent pterygoidal process.
- Short, lordotic skull base.
- A narrow, posteriorly rotated protuberant facial skeleton with shallow externally oblique orbits.
- All calvarial bones are present but are small and deformed.
- Absence of anterior and middle cranial fossa with anteriorly placed tympanic rings with transverse presence of temporal bones.
- Palatal abnormalities present.

## Musculoskeletal extremities

- Deficient ribs, ulna with vertebral anomalies.
- Contracture of fingers with cervical rachischisis.
- Club feet (talipes equino varus).
- Multiple contractures called *arthrogryposis multiplex congenita*.
- Infants with anencephaly have been shown to have lower limb movement on ultrasonography.

## Cardiorespiratory system

- 5% of cases present with cardiovascular anomalies.
- Lungs are small due to lack of breathing effort but show epithelial and biochemical maturation appropriate for the gestational age.
- Evidence of aspiration of neural elements from amniotic fluid has been reported.

## Gastrointestinal system

• Liver and kidney with lighter weights have been demonstrated.

## Endocrine system

• Total absence of hypothalamus with presence of anterior pituitary (amount of pituitary gland varies).
• Presence of posterior pituitary in one quarter of cases.
• Endocrinological studies demonstrated the presence of prolactin and thyroid stimulating hormone (TSH). However, there is a lack of adrenocorticotropic hormone (ACTH), resulting in hypoplasia of fetal adrenal cortex.
• Thyroid gland and islets of Langerhans are normal.

## Differential diagnosis

• Iniencephaly
• Cranioectodermal hypoplasia

### *Explanation*

• Iniencephaly vs. anencephaly: In iniencephaly, a cranial cavity is present with skin covering the head and the retroflexed region.
• Cranioectodermal hypoplasia: Calvarial bones are absent with cephalad bony structure, whereas in anencephaly calvarial bones are present but deformed.

## Survival of Anencephalic Infants: Role of Ethics

Survival of anencephalic infants depends on degree of brain stem dysgenesis and the medical and nursing care. Although incompatible with survival beyond a few days, reports of survival up to 14 months have been reported. Trauma during the process of labor can result in damage to brain stem with secondary hypoventilation and cardiorespiratory arrest.

Those infants whose brain stem functions are intact succumb to severe endocrine deficiency with secondary electrolyte abnormalities. Cardiac arrhythmia is also a cause of death. Infection is a rare cause of death as most cases die before infection can set in. For those rare cases of infants with anencephaly surviving months, the commonest cause of death is aspiration.

## Suggested Readings

Baird P, Sadovnick A. Survival in infants with anencephaly. *Clin Pediatr* (*Phila*) 1984; **23**:268.

Blanco Muñoz J, Lacasaña M, Borja Aburto VH, Torres Sánchez LE, García García AM, López Carrillo L. Socioeconomic factors and the risk of anencephaly in a Mexican population: A case-control study. *Public Health Rep* 2005 Jan–Feb; **120**(1):39–45.

Dias MS, Partington M. Embryology of myelomeningocele and anencephaly. *Neurosurg Focus* 2004; **16**(2): Article 1.

Metzner L, Garol JD, Fields HW Jr, Kokich VG. The craniofacial skeleton in anencephalic human fetuses ill. Facial skeleton. *Teratology* 1978; **17**(1):75–82.

Müller F, O'Rahilly R. Development of anencephaly and its variants. *Amer J Anat* 1991; **190**:193–218.

Shewmon D, Anencephaly: Selected medical aspects. Hastings Center Report October/ November 1988.

Vieira AR, Castillo Taucher S. Maternal age and neural tube defects: Evidence for a greater effect in spina bifida than in anencephaly. *Rev Med Chil* 2005; **133**(1):62–70. Epub 2005 Mar 10.

# Chapter 21

# Iniencephaly

## Definition

Iniencephaly has three main distinguishing features:

- Deficit in the occipital bone that result in an enlarged foramen magnum.
- Incomplete or irregular fusion of the cervical and thoracic vertebral arches and bodies.
- Hyperextension of the malformed cervicothoracic spine with upturned face due to marked lordosis.

Some consider iniencephaly as a severe form of Klippel–Feil deformity. Chiari type III has also been associated with iniencephaly.

Iniencephaly is one of the rarest forms of neural tube defects, presenting with rachischisis involving the nape of the neck and the occiput, hence the name which comes from the Greek word *Inion*, meaning "nape of the neck". Iniencephaly is almost completely lethal, with only six cases reported to survive for a long term.

## Historical Perspective

Saint-Hilaire was the first one to describe a case of iniencephaly in 1836. He proposed that it is caused by arrest of the embryo in physiological retroflexion of the head during the third week of gestation or by the failure of normal forward bending during the fourth week.

H.L. Lewis in 1897 described iniencephaly to be a rachischisis of the cervical spine and retroflexion of the head. He also classified iniencephaly into two categories: one associated with encephalocele called *iniencephaly apertus* and the other without encephalocele called *iniencephalus clausus*.

## Incidence and Prevalence

- A very rare disorder with an incidence of 0.1 in 10,000 live births to 1 in 65,000 live births.
- Female fetuses have a higher incidence than male fetuses, female to male ratio is 9:1.
- True incidence is underestimated as most fetuses are stillborn.

## Molecular Genetics

Recurrence rate is less than 1% but may be higher, up to 5% in families with a history of neural tube defect.

## Pathogenesis

Pathogenesis of this rare neural tube defect is not exactly known.

- Most theories try to explain this rare neural tube defect as a primary neural anomaly. It was Marin-Padilla who stated that mesoderm insufficiency is the root cause of the anomaly.
- The main pathophysiology of the defect is anomaly of the occipital bone combined with raschischisis, i.e. non-fused spine. The remainder is just simple herniation of cranial contents during the gestational period.

## Embryological Theories

Warkany *et al.* hypothesized that iniencephaly is resulted from arrest of physiological retroflexion that takes place in an embryo during the third week of gestation period.

## Possible etiological agents

- Maternal infections like syphilis
- Drugs such as clomiphene citrate
- Antibiotics such as sulphonamide and tetracycline

## Clinical Manifestations and Diagnostic Imaging

- Most cases are stillborn and compatibility with life is depended on severity of associated malformations and degree of retroflexion.
- Up to date only six long-term survivors are known.

## Associated malformations

- Urinary anomalies are the most frequent accompanying anomalies seen.
- Gastrointestinal followed by cardiovascular involvement is the next most common associated anomaly with a frequency of 8% reported in each case.

## Most frequent single malformations

- Hydronephrosis (8%)
- Cleft palate (8%)
- Diaphragmatic hernia (5%)
- Exophthalmos (5%)
- Horseshoe kidney (4%)

## Other associated anomalies

### CNS

- Spina bifida is the most common anomaly with 50% of cases being reported
- Holoprosencephaly
- Agyria
- Lissencephaly
- Cyclopia
- Dandy–Walker malformation or dysplastic cerebellum

### Craniofacial

- Cleft palate/cleft lip

- Absence of mandible
- Low-set ears

*Gastrointestinal anomalies*

- Diaphragmatic hernia/agenesis
- Omphalocele
- Gastroschisis
- Gastrointestinal tract atresia

*Cardiothoracic anomalies*

- Congenital heart disease such as ventricular septal defect (VSD) or atrial septal defect (ASD)
- Pulmonary hypoplasia

*Placental anomalies*

- Single umbilical artery
- Chromosomal abnormalities like trophoblastic inclusions
- Retroplacental hematoma

## Antenatal Diagnosis

Ultrasonography is still the best initial diagnostic methodology for screening neural tube defect.

Some diagnostic features include:

- Exaggerated lordosis to the extent that neck is missing
- Raschischisis
- Imperfect formation of skull base at foramen magnum
- Variable fusion of inion with cervicothoracic spine and resultant severe dorsiflexion of head

## Suggested Readings

David TJ, Nixon A. Congenital malformations associated with anencephaly and inien-cephaly. *J Med Genet* 1976; **13**:263–265.

de Jong TH. Deliberate termination of life of newborns with spina bifida, a critical reappraisal. *Child's Nerv Syst* 2008; **24**(1):13–28; discussion 29–56. Epub 2007 Oct 10.

Erdinçler P, Kaynar MY, Canbaz B, Koçer N, Kuday C, Ciplak N. Iniencephaly: Neuroradiological and surgical features. *J Neurosurg* 1998; **89**:317–320.

Gartman JJ, Melin TE, Lawrence WT. Deformity correction and long-term survival in an infant with iniencephaly. *J Neurosurg* 1991; **75**:126–130.

Katz VL, Aylsworth AS, Albright SG. Iniencephaly is not uniformly fatal. *Prenat Diagn* 1989; **9**:595–599.

Munden MM, Macpherson RI, Cure J. Iniencephaly: 3D-computed tomography imaging. *Pediatr Radiol* 1993; **23**:572.

Paterson SJ. Iniencephalus. *J Obstet Gynaecol Br Emp* 1944; **51**:330–333.

Rodriguez MM, Reik RA, Carreno TD. Cluster of iniencephaly in Miami. *Pediatr Pathol* 1991; **11**:211–221.

## Chapter 22

# Encephalocele

## Introduction

The encephalocele is one of the most challenging conditions for the patients, their families and the treating physicians. As the malformation affects the skull, children with this condition are more easily stigmatized than children affected with spinal defects, albeit the latter are more disabling.

## Definition

In essence, an encephalocele is defined as protrusion of a portion of the brain through a defect in the skull. The content of an encephalocele sac may vary. When there is only brain parenchyma in the encephalocele sac, it is called *cephalocele*; when there is presence of a large cystic component without the presence of any brain tissue and is covered with meningeal covering, it is called *meningocele*. If the contents of the sac have part of the ventricle along with the abovementioned contents then it is called a *ventriculocele*. However, throughout this text, the term *encephalocele* is used for all lesions with herniation of cranial contents.

## Historical Perspective

Encephalocele is the cranial counterpart of spinal dysraphism called *cranium bifidum*. It was Geoffrey Saint-Hilaire who was the first to describe and name this anomaly as "Notencephale" in 1820.

## Epidemiology

- Incidence of encephalocele: 0.8 to 5.6 per 10,000 births.
- Encephalocele account for 10–20% of neural tube defects.
- 70% of occipital encephalocele are seen in females.

• **Geographic variation**: Encephalocele incidence has been observed to have a variable geographic distribution. The reason behind this variation is yet to be defined. In Europe and America, occipital encephalocele is the most common form of encephalocele as compared to the Southeast Asian countries like Thailand, Malaysia, northern India, Myanmar and Russia, where anterior encephalocele is the predominant type of encephalocele.

## Pathogenesis

Encephaloceles are multifactorial in origin with various genetic and environmental factors involved. Some potential teratogens implicated in the pathogenesis of encephalocele are as follows:

• Gestational hyperthermia
• Synthetic vitamin A, used commonly as an antiacne agent in the first trimester
• Cholesterol lowering drugs like clofibrate
• Antiepileptic agent like primidone which are folic acid antagonist

   The fact that encephalocele are always covered by full-thickness skin and membranes lead embryologists to theorize that the defect in encephalocele must have arisen after closure of the neural tube. This observation makes encephalocele a distinct lesion from its spinal counterpart, myelomeningocele, which arises due to aberration during primary neurulation. Hence, encephalocele can be grouped under a broader umbrella term called *postneurulation defects*. A typical feature of this postneurulation defect is failure of bony fusion in the midline with subsequent herniation of the cranial contents. However, this hypothesis needs further conformation and it is left to the readers to pursue further reading of the embryological theories of such congenital malformations.

   Controversy exists in connection with ingestion of folic acid and its influence on the incidence rate of encephalocele. From various studies it has been noted that folic acid has little, if any, impact on reducing the incidence of encephalocele, although there has been remarkable decrease in the incidence rate of anencephaly and myelomeningocele. This indicates that there is probably a different mechanism involved in the pathogenesis of encephalocele which is distinct from its spinal counterpart.

## Classification

### Modified classification by Rosenfeld and Watters

1. **Convexity encephalocele**

   - Occipital
   - Parietal
   - Occipitocervical

2. **Sincipital/Anterior**

   - Frontoethmoidal
   - Interfrontal
   - Craniofacial cleft

3. **Basal**

   - Transsphenoidal
   - Spheno-orbital
   - Transethmoidal
   - Sphenoethmoidal

4. **Atretic**

### Surgical classification

A lesion that has attracted the attention of so many researchers has led to many classifications. Acknowledging that they are useful and accurate we will opt for the one that is commonly used by craniofacial surgeons and pediatric neurosurgeons in clinical practice. The description of encephalocele will be written following this classification.

- Basal
- Anterior (also called frontal)
- Occipital
- Parietal

## Prognostic Factors in Encephalocele

The clinical outcome of a child with encephalocele can be predicted approximately by the following characteristics:

- Site of the defect
- Size of the sac and associated microcephaly

- Presence of brain parenchyma in the encephalocele sac
- Associated cerebral anomalies like agenesis of corpus callosum
- Development of seizures

It has been observed that anterior encephalocele has a better clinical outcome than posterior encephalocele in terms of neurocognitive development. However, as we go through the following section, it will be evident that even though children afflicted with anterior encephalocele achieve good neurocognitive development, it has many associated medical comorbidities like hormonal imbalance.

## Basal encephalocele

### Definition

Herniation of brain parenchyma through a defect in the anterior skull base either through the cribriform plate or the sphenoid bone is called *basal encephalocele*. They are rare, with some variants going unnoticed right up to adulthood when they are discovered by diligent ENT specialists. These encephalocele are thought to arise from an aberration which affects the growth of the base of the skull or the chondrocranium before the tenth week of gestation.

The image below shows the encephalocele protruding through the cleft palate of a ten-year-old boy with past history of cleft lip repaired at one year of age and an unrepaired cleft palate. Presence of true hypertelorism and horizontal dystopia with blind right eye and bifid nose are also noted.

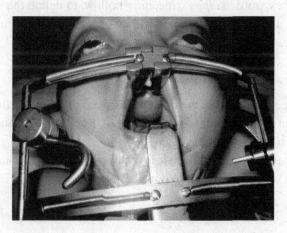

MRI report shows a large defect in frontoethmoidal bone extending from the posterior ethmoid air cells into the oral cavity through a defect in the palate. The encephalocele measures $43 \times 40$ mm in size. There is no brain parenchyma in the sac.

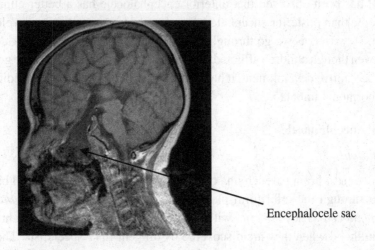

Encephalocele sac

### Associated features

Anterior lobe of pituitary is not well formed. Right globe is proptotic with atrophic right optic nerve. There is agenesis of corpus callosum with presence of colpocephaly. When occipital horns are larger and wider than normal sized frontal horns, it is called *colpocephaly*. The term comes from the Greek word "*kolpos*", meaning hollow, to define the same brain abnormality, and described as a persistence of fetal cerebral ventricles into postnatal life.

### Epidemiology of basal encephalocele

- Basal encephalocele are the rarest form among the encephalocele, with a reported incidence of 1 in 35,000 to 40,000 live births and accounts for only 10% of all encephalocele.
- Among basal encephaloceles, it is the transsphenoidal variant which is the rarest of all, with a reported incidence of probably 1 in 700,000 live

births. This variant is mentioned separately because it is commonly associated with hormonal imbalance. Thus the more posterior the encephalocele is, the rarer is its incidence.

• No gender preference is observed.

## Embryogenesis of basal encephalocele

The general acceptance is that of an aberration affecting the development of bones of the anterior skull base, called the *chondrocranium*. The gestational period corresponding to this deficiency is usually before the tenth week of intrauterine life. The various theories explaining this anomaly are mentioned as follows:

### Theory of failure of closure of anterior neuropore

One of the earliest theories postulated by Mood *et al.* states that the primary defect in the evolution of basal encephalocele is non-separation of neuroectoderm from surface ectoderm at the cephalic end of the embryo, due to failure of closure of the anterior neuropore at the end of fourth week of gestation.

This secondarily resulted in failure of the mesodermal primordial cells (which will give rise to future skull bones) from penetrating between the two ectodermal layers. Thus, there is an area deficient in bony covering and instead the neuroectodermal cells of the developing diencephalic vesicle remain in contact with the cutaneous ectoderm of the primitive oral cavity. At times partial fusion of the bony covering will lead to a sequestered encephalocele or cerebral heterotopia which has lost its connection with the subarachnoid space and is called *atretic encephalocele*.

Subsequent growth of the diencephalic vesicle will in turn lead to abnormal development of the neighboring segments of neuraxis and its coverings. This will manifest as associated cerebral malformations accompanying basal encephalocele such as agenesis of corpus callosum, abnormalities of optic chiasma and tract, and anomalies of the skull base bones.

Although the theory is still well accepted, we will discuss other possible hypotheses regarding embryogenesis of basal encephalocele.

*Theory of primary bony defect*

Primary bony defect manifesting as secondary failure of ossification and chondrification of the anterior skull base around the sphenoid bone can lead to bony defects with subsequent herniation of intracranial structures, resulting in basal encephalocele (enchondral ossification or chondrification, meaning ossification of bone from a cartilage).

*Theory of reopening of closed neural tube*

Localized increase in intracranial pressure with secondary reopening of the closed or fused anterior neural tube.

*Theory of persistence of craniopharyngeal canal*

The persistence of craniopharyngeal canal, which is the embryological path of migration of the Rathke's pouch and which usually closes by the 50th day of embryonic life, will probably explain the transphenoidal variant of basal encephalocele with secondary herniation of intracranial structures like hypophysis, anterior part of the third ventricle, optic chiasma and optic nerves.

*Classification by topographical localization*

The most widely accepted classification of basal encephalocele is based on anatomical position of the herniation. This classification is by Suwanwela and Suwanwela in 1972. In 1987, Nager *et al.* added another variant to the present classification, which is the sphenomaxillary form.

1. **Transsphenoidal**: Defect in the body or wings of sphenoid through which sac protrudes into the nasopharynx or occupies the sphenoid sinus without protruding. Thus there are two types of transsphenoidal encephalocele: *intrasphenoidal*, which is extension into the sphenoid sinus and *true transsphenoidal*, which is extension beyond the sphenoid sinus into the nasal cavity or the nasopharynx.
2. **Sphenoethmoidal**: Herniation of cranial contents into the posterior portion of nasal cavity exiting through posterior portion of nasal roof secondary to imperfect union or widening of sphenoethmoidal suture.
3. **Transethmoidal**: Exit through bony defect in cribriform plate in the anterior portion of nasal fossa.

4. **Spheno-orbital**: Exit through superior orbital fissure and cause exoph-thalmoses.
5. **Sphenomaxillary**: This encephalocele was added to the group of basal encephalocele by Nager *et al.* The lesion exits through the inferior orbital fissure to the pterygopalatine fossa.

*Clinical presentation*

The clinical manifestations of basal encephalocele are variable, with cases going unnoticed right up to adulthood when it is detected due to non-related clinical symptoms like seizures or nasal obstruction. However, there are two distinct dysmorphic features which can serve as clues to the underlying cranial defect in infants and they are as follows:

• Broad nasal root with hypertelorism
• Increased bitemporal diameter

Basal encephalocele has also been addressed in the literature as "*long nose hypertelorism syndrome*", where hypertelorism means increased dis-tance between the two eyes along with a broad nasal root. This term has become obsolete and to avoid any confusion, we have retained the term basal encephalocele throughout the text.

Depending on the site of herniation, basal encephalocele can be in the nasal cavity (transethmoidal or sphenoethmoidal), the nasopharynx, the sphenoid sinus (sphenoethmoidal or transsphenoidal), the orbits (spheno-orbital) or the sphenomaxillary fossa (sphenomaxillary). The clinical presentations vary accordingly and are explained under the following headings:

1. Craniofacial abnormalities
2. Presence of a nasal or pharyngeal mass
3. Ocular defects
4. Endocrine defects
5. CSF rhinorrhea and recurrent meningitis
6. Associated intracranial anomalies

The clinical description of basal encephalocele can also be based on the age of presentation.

i. *Early onset symptoms*
   Presence of dysmorphic features along with complaints of respiratory
   obstruction from nasal or pharyngeal mass, apnea or respiratory distress,
   or symptoms dominated by feeding difficulties and failure to thrive are
   symptoms of encephalocele that can be detected early. Occasionally
   there may be accompanying seizures seen with intracranial malformations and basilar meningitis from CSF leaks.

ii. *Late onset symptoms*
   Those basal encephaloceles which escape early diagnosis and remain
   asymptomatic right up to adolescent or even adulthood are detected most
   commonly by ENT specialists due to symptoms like nasal obstruction
   mimicking nasal polyp. Many occult basal encephalocele present with
   basilar meningitis caused by the sinus flora. This gives clue to possible
   patent connection between the intranasal and intracranial spaces resulting in the diagnosis of basal encephalocele. Rarely hormonal imbalance
   is the presenting complaint. With this in mind we continue with the
   details of each clinical presentation.

1. **Craniofacial abnormalities**: During infancy, presence of obvious
craniofacial defects such as true orbital hypertelorism, cleft lip and cleft
palate leads to the diagnosis of the underlying skull base defect.

- *True orbital hypertelorism*
  Hypertelorism, which means increased distance between the two eye-
  balls, is due to increased distance between the medial and the lateral walls
  of the orbit. True hypertelorism is seen along with basal encephalocele.
  Pseudohypertelorism is only seen when the distance between the medial
  walls of the orbit are increased as in sincipital encephalocele.
- *Cleft lip and cleft palate*
  Cleft lip and cleft palate are part of orofacial clefts which arise due to
  failure of the maxillary process to fuse with the frontonasal process.
  Incidentally, orofacial clefts are also seen frequently in folic acid
  deficiency states. Presence of frontonasal dysplasia with either broad
  nasal root or bifid nose is also observed.

2. **Presence of a nasal or pharyngeal mass**: The presence of a nasal or pharyngeal mass presenting with the following symptoms can lead to early diagnosis of basal encephalocele:

- Nasal obstruction
- Respiratory difficulties with apneic spells
- Feeding difficulties leading to failure to thrive
- Alteration of voice

Clinical findings of mass in the nasopharynx :

- *Midline mass covered by mucosa*
- *Pulsatile mass and increases in size upon crying or Valsalva maneuver*
  Pulsatility and increase in size of mass upon Valsalva maneuver or crying in children indicate patent communication with the intracranial compartment.
- *Positive Furstenberg test*
  Increase in size of mass in the nasopharynx on pressure over the ipsilateral jugular veins is called the *Furstenberg sign*. In children, the sign is manifested when the child strains or cries. It is an additional confirmation sign of basal encephalocele that indicates a connection with the intracranial compartment. With the advent of MRI imaging, which is the diagnostic investigation of choice for evaluation of the encephalocele, these clinical signs have become obsolete. Nevertheless the importance of Furstenberg test in the pre-MRI era cannot be undermined.

Differential diagnosis: When faced with a mass in the nasopharynx, the treating physicians should be able to differentiate:

- Basal encephalocele
- Enlarged adenoids

There have been cases reported where basal encephalocele was mistaken for an adenoid and was operated on, resulting invariably in a fatal outcome.

3. **Ocular defects**: The spheno-orbital variant presents with the following ocular defects which can be detected in infants or older children complaining of visual defects:

   i. Fixed or progressive visual loss
  ii. Strabismus or squint
 iii. Congenital optic disc anomalies like morning glory syndrome and coloboma of optic neural head

*Morning glory syndrome*

This is a type of optic disc anomaly which clinically presents as decreased visual acuity. On fundoscopy examination, the optic disc appears enlarged and funnel-shaped with a central white dot, which is the glial tissue and this is surrounded by an annulus of chorioretinal pigmentary disturbance, giving it an appearance just like that of a morning glory flower (tropical flower). Defective closure of fetal optic fissure during embryonic development leads to optic nerve dysplasia.

*Coloboma of optic neural head*

Coloboma is a congenital optic disc anomaly where the disc appears deeply excavated on fundus examination while the patient presents with visual field defects.

4. **Endocrine defects**: Endocrine defects are detected in older children when one of the following signs of hormonal imbalance is evident:

- Delayed puberty
- Diabetes insipidus
- Short stature

Endocrine profiles of these children most commonly reveal hypogonadotrophic hypogonadism and central diabetes insipidus, indicating mostly hypothalamic origin of hormonal dysfunction rather than pituitary dysfunction. However, a combined picture is not uncommon. Possible mechanisms underlying the hormonal defects are thought to arise from either of the following conditions:

- Primary hypothalamic-pituitary dysgenesis
- Secondary degeneration or atrophy of pituitary-hypothalamic connections from mechanical distortion by the encephalocele

Basal encephalocele should be suspected when the triad of hypertelorism (ophthalmic complaints, endocrine abnormalities and presence of nasopharyngeal mass) are present in a child.

5. **CSF rhinorrhea and recurrent meningitis**: When a child presents with basilar meningitis, its usual clinical presentation of lower cranial nerve deficits involve most commonly the facial nerve. Possible causes of basilar meningitis in a child are Lyme disease or tuberculous meningitis, both very rare cases. However, recurrent meningitis, clear nasal discharge, nasal obstruction and headaches after blowing of nose, all points towards a patent ascending route to the intracranial compartment, giving clues to a diagnosis of basal encephalocele. The most common pathogenic organism causing recurrent meningitis is *Streptococcus pneumonia*, which is present in the nasal flora.

6. **Associated intracranial anomalies**: The following are types of associated cerebral malformations commonly seen with basal encephalocele.

- Agenesis of corpus callosum (ACC)
- Mild mental retardation and hydrocephalus

Patients with ACC exhibit a pattern of delayed motor development, difficulty with balance and bilateral hand movement deficits, large head size, poor muscle tone, poor depth and reduced pain perception. Interestingly, not every child with ACC will present with the full gamut of symptoms. Nonetheless, it is important to remember that the mechanism of the diseases is not limited to what we can detect. Similarly, it could be intuitive to associate the defects of the oropharynx and the visual system, which are a constant feature in these patients with encephalocele; but considering that the hard palate and the visual system are developed around the same time we should consider the possibility that cleft palate, visual impairment (e.g. morning glory syndrome) and agenesis of the corpus callosum are actually a yet unnamed pathology.

*Diagnostic imaging*

With the clinical suspicion of presence of a basal encephalocele, the treating physician should evaluate the patient with the following investigations:

- CT scan brain with 3D reconstruction

- MRI brain and MR angiography

An associated MR angiography helps to identify any vascular anomaly and delineate the vascular anatomy in relation with the basal encephalocele. These points will help in surgical planning to repair the skull defect.

*Ancillary investigations*

- Ophthalmic evaluation
- Hormonal profile

*Common differential diagnosis of nasal mass*

As a continuation of the above discussion, the readers are now aware of the fact that basal encephalocele presents in the adolescent age mostly with complaints that are recognized by ENT specialist. Here we explain the common differentials for a nasal mass which can range from a benign nasal polyp to an encephalocele.

|  | Encephalocele | Nasal glioma | Dermoid cyst | Nasal polyp |
|---|---|---|---|---|
| Age | <5 years | <5 years | Any | >5 years |
| Location | Variable | Variable | Variable | Intranasal |
| Pulsation | Yes | — | — | — |
| Variable size | Yes | — | — | — |
| Cranial defect | Yes | Rare | Rare | No |

**Note on nasal glioma**:

- This is a misnomer as it is not a neoplasm at all.
- Nasal glioma is an encephalocele that becomes sequestered from the brain and cranial vault, is associated with early degeneration of the stalk and has lost its connection with the subarachnoid space.
- Nasal glioma is a differential form of basal encephalocele.

*Natural history*

The lesion has an unpredictable course where it can present early in life as illustrated in this clinical report or may remain asymptomatic till adolescence when the clinical presentations include hormonal imbalance,

visual problem or even recurrent meningitis. Nonetheless, as illustrated by
the two cases below, the mode of presentation encompasses a large array
of symptoms and depend on the patient's demographics.

A baby with unilateral cleft lip, midline cleft palate and hypertelorism
developed meningitis in the first 48 hours of life. Examination of the
nasopharynx showed a soft tissue mass, which was confirmed as a basal
encephalocele by computed tomography. There was associated presence
of congenital hydrocephalus and absence of corpus callosum. Surgical
treatment included repair of the anterior basal skull defect, repair of the cleft
lip and cleft palate, followed by placement of a ventriculoperitoneal shunt.
From recent clinical evaluation of the child, there is evidence of developmental delay and visual impairment due to morning glory syndrome in the
right eye. This case demonstrates that basal encephalocele should be considered in any baby with midline facial deformity and recurrent meningitis.

A 52-year-old female presented with a two-day history of headaches,
pyrexia (38°C), neck stiffness and photophobia. Three days prior to this
she also described spontaneous discharge of clear fluid from her right
nostril. This clinical scenario can be explained by the fact that the lady had
presented with CSF leakage through the nose, known as *CSF rhinorrhea* and
subsequent development of meningitis. This depicts another spectrum of
clinical presentation of basal encephalocele. However, regardless of the age
of presentation of basal encephalocele, all such lesions should be referred
to competent neurosurgical services. We acknowledge that this may pose a
problem for developing nations; nonetheless it will still be a responsibility
of the treating physicians to advocate for their patient's well-being.

## Surgery

The goal of surgical repair is to prevent infections like meningitis and
to decrease any respiratory obstruction. Correction of hypertelorism and
strabismus are important aspects of the management process as they have an
impact on the quality of life of the affected children. The sac is approached
intradurally through a subfrontal craniotomy. The close relation between
the root of the encephalocele, the pituitary hypothalamic stalk and the
optic apparatus needs to be acknowledged when deciding the best surgical
approach. Recently it is a common practice to "push" the sac up from below,

from the oropharynx. In this approach, the risk of meningitis is substantially diminished. A single surgery performed by a team of neurosurgeons and craniofacial surgeons is the gold standard of treatment planning.

## Sincipital encephalocele

### Definition

The protrusion of brain parenchyma through a defect in the frontoethmoidal junction, or between the frontal process of the maxilla and nasal bone is called *sincipital encephalocele*. The most common defect lies at the foramen caecum (frontal bone) and the crista galli (ethmoid) which forms the posterior margin of the defect. The herniated content may be unilateral, bilateral or midline structures with little correlation between the volume of the content and the diameter of the skull defect.

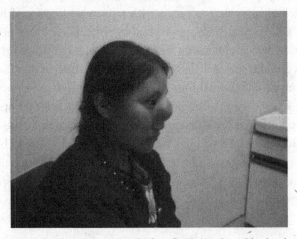

This image shows the picture of a young girl from South America, with a basal encephalocele.

Two distinct pathological conditions which have similar presentations are described here:

- Primary sincipital encephalocele
- Secondary sincipital encephalocele

The primary sincipital encephalocele represents a neural tube defect and this will be the main subject of our discussion here. The secondary sincipital encephalocele is a rare clinical entity which is associated primarily with craniofacial clefts like cleft lip and cleft palate with secondary herniation of cranial contents. The elaboration of these defects is covered in texts of craniofacial defects and thus will not be included in our text.

A nine-month-old male presents with mass in front of right orbit.

*MRI*:

- Defect in anterior skull base adjacent to cribriform plate measuring $5 \times 9$ mm.
- Herniation of right orbitofrontal gyrus into the medial aspect of right orbit, which is partly cystic.
- The cystic component of the herniating tissue is displacing the right medial rectus muscle laterally and the right lamina papyracea medially with lateral displacement of right globe.
- The images below are consistent with sincipital encephalocele (naso-orbital variant).

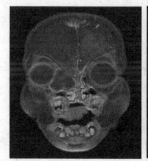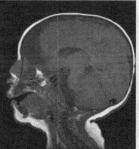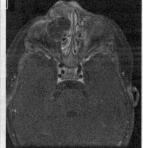

A five-year-old child presents with massive nasofrontal encephalocele. The neuroradiologist describes the presence of an anterior encephalocele with distortion and dilation of frontal horn of right lateral ventricle. The corpus callosum is thinned and elongated. Presence of some interdigitations are also noted in the medial aspects of frontal and parietal lobes, suggesting falcine hypoplasia. The herniated anterior frontal lobes appear to have some volume loss with increased flair signal intensity consistent with encephalomalacia.

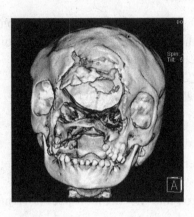
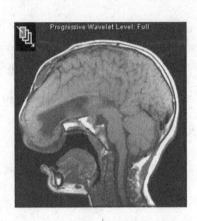

There is no doubt that sincipital (frontal for short) encephaloceles are a formidable problem for the affected children and their families. In contrast to other variants of occipital encephaloceles, the survival rate of the sincipital encephaloceles is very high. The lesion is away from the brain stem and causes minimal impact on the pituitary, but the facial deformity and the subsequent stigma is powerful enough to prompt the physicians to take action or to prompt the families to hide the affected children away from public eye.

## Historical perspective

J. Weber *et al.* from Berlin Museum of Medical History, Germany, reported a deformed skull belonging to an approximately 45-year-old woman from the 16th century, from the province of Salta (Calchaqui), located at the north of Argentina. The skull defect was consistent with frontoethmoidal encephalocele. The skull is now part of the Rudolf Virchow collection in Berlin (Berlin Museum of Medical History, Department of Historical Anthropology) and carries the repository ID "S4882".

In 1972, extensive work on sincipital encephalocele had been undertaken by Suwanwela *et al.* from Thailand. Incidentally, Thailand has the highest incidence rate of sincipital encephalocele in the world.

## Incidence and prevalence

- In western countries, the incidence is 1 in 35,000 live births, which are rarer than the more common occipital encephalocele seen in Caucasian infants.

- A high incidence of sincipital encephalocele is seen in Southeast Asian countries like Thailand, Indonesia, Myanmar, Malaysia, Northern India and Russia, with the highest incidence reported from Thailand (1 in 5000 live births).
- There is equal distribution among gender.
- Among the sincipital encephaloceles, the frontoethmoidal form is the most common.
- Hydrocephalus is uncommon among anterior encephalocele with a reported incidence of 10–15% only. However, deficits in neurocognitive development are rarely encountered in anterior encephalocele as compared to the posterior encephalocele.

### Inheritance pattern

No familial cases have been reported in sincipital encephalocele.

### Syndromes associated with sincipital encephalocele

Most sincipital encephalocele arise without any associated syndromes, yet there are case reports of occurrence of the following syndromic encephaloceles which one rarely encounters in the clinical setting:

## Craniofacial defects

- *Apert syndrome*
  Apert syndrome has two distinct features, bicoronal synostosis and maxillary hypoplasia, which is clinically seen as midfacial hypoplasia. The other craniofacial deformities seen in Apert syndrome are hypertelorism, exophthalmoses or proptosis and antimongoloid eyes, or laterally down-sloping slant of eyes. Low-set ears accompanied by an abnormally small, flat nasal structure with a bulbous tip and syndactyly are common clinically detected features.
- *Goldenhar syndrome*
  Oculo-auriculo-vertebral (OAV) syndrome or Goldenhar syndrome is a congenital disorder affecting the CNS, cardiac and renal system. It is thought to arise from dysplasia of the first and second branchial arches. Clinically it presents as facial microsomia and ocular epibulbar dermoid. The nervous system manifestations of this syndrome include

encephalocele, spina bifida, cervical vertebral fusion, hemivertebrae and scoliosis.

- *HARD + E syndrome*, which is constellation of the following conditions:
  H — hydrocephalus
  A — agyria
  RD — retinal dysplasia
  E — encephalocele

## Classification based on anatomical location

### i. Frontoethmoidal

**Nasoethmoidal**: defect between lamina cribosa and ethmoidal bone.
**Nasofrontal**: defect in bregmatic region between two deformed orbits with orifice above the ethmoid.
**Naso-orbital**: defect at junction of ethmoid and frontal process of maxilla.

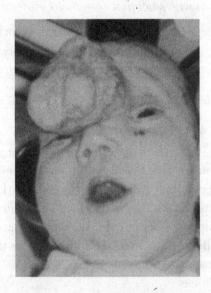

### ii. Interfrontal
In the image above we observe a frontal sac that respects the anatomy of the nasal bones, thus it is not typically nasofrontal.

### iii. Craniofacial cleft

## Classification based on severity

**Type I**: There is lateral displacement of medial wall of orbit, i.e. the medial canthus of eye and is called *pseudo-hypertelorism* along with lacrimal duct obstruction.

**Type II**: Superior displacement of the eyebrow and inferior displacement of the nasal tip, known as *long nose deformity*.

**Type III**: Presence of true hypertelorism manifesting as increased distance between the medial and the lateral walls of the orbit.

## Embryology

There are a series of theories that might explain anterior encephalocele.

### Defective closure of rostral neuropore theory

Rostral neuropore closes in a bidirectional fashion starting from the rhombencephalon in caudorostral direction and from chiasmatic plate in rostrocaudal direction. This process takes place around the third week of gestational period. The site of final bidirectional closure is situated between nasal fields and corresponds with a midline skull defect at the foramen caecum. This is thus the primary site of all defects associated with anterior or sincipital encephalocele.

Any disturbance at this site would result in persistent connection between neuroectoderm (brain) and surface ectoderm (skin). Disturbance in final closure of the rostral neuropore could be due to incomplete apoptotic process, resulting in secondary persistent connection between neuroectoderm and surface ectoderm. This disturbance could secondarily lead to failure of formation of intermediate mesodermal tissue (skull bones), secondarily result in a defect in the skull bones with subsequent herniation of brain tissue, developing into an encephalocele.

### Defective tissular induction with malformation early in embryogenesis of membranous cranial roof

According to this theory, abnormal development and ossification of the calvarial bones is the fundamental defect causing encephalocele. The membranous roof of cranial cavity is present between the 38th and 40th day of gestation period. The first two ossification centers in the frontal bone appear between the 50th and 60th day of embryonic life, in the region of future superciliary arches. Intramembranous ossification starts at these two centers and eventually spreads dorsally over the pars orbitalis in the direction of sphenoid and ethmoid bones. The union of these two ossification centers is at the midline where the metopic suture persists.

There is a weak spot in the anterior skull base where the frontal and the ethmoidal bones meet. The presence of this weak spot can be explained by the fact that the frontal bone ossifies by membranous ossification, as compared to the ethmoid bones which undergo endochondral ossification. Thus a defect in the ossification process can lead to anomalous bony development of anterior skull base.

## Possible etiological agents or teratogens

Exposure to any of these agents in the first trimester can increase the risk of developing encephalocele:

- Vitamin A
- Trypan A
- X-ray irradiation

## Clinical manifestations

As compared to the previously described basal encephalocele, sincipital encephaloceles are diagnosed at a much earlier age, most commonly in infancy due to presence of more obvious facial defects.

## Common clinical signs

i.  Swelling or mass over nose or inner canthus
ii. Ophthalmic complaints
iii. Neurological issues

i.  *Swelling or mass over nose or inner canthus*
    On examination of the mass, the following signs are observed:

    - Globular mass
    - Compressible and fluctuation test positive
    - Covered with skin, usually with skin showing scarring or thickening

- Superficial ulceration present in a minority of cases
- Transillumination test positive
- Expandable swelling on Valsalva maneuver

**Furstenberg test**: Increase in size of mass on pressure over the jugular veins most commonly seen in infants while crying is called the *Furstenberg test*. However, in this era of MRI imaging, this clinical test is no longer elucidated. This sign indicates communication with the intracranial compartment and has been mentioned in the previous section.

ii. *Ophthalmic complaints*

- Telecanthus is characteristic of sincipital encephalocele and is clinically detected as wide-set eyes. Most patients have a medial intercanthal distance greater than 97th percentile
- Eyes are proptosed/dystopic or absent
- Presence of strabismus and hypertelorism
- Lacrimal drainage dysfunction with epiphora, i.e. tearing of eyes

**A short note on hypertelorism seen with sincipital encephalocele**: Sincipital encephalocele is associated with interorbital hypertelorism, which is increased distance only between the medial walls of the orbit and is called *pseudo-hypertelorism*. This anomaly results secondarily from any disturbance in the development of frontoethmoidal complex. This is in contrast to basal encephalocele where there is presence of true hypertelorism, defined as increased distance between the medial and the lateral orbital walls. The defect arises from the failure of medialization of the entire orbital walls.

iii. *Neurological signs and symptoms*

- Infection: recurrent meningitis or abscess
- Epilepsy
- Hydrocephalus
- Developmental delay or mental retardation
- Agenesis of corpus callosum
- Intracerebral lipoma

*Diagnostic imaging*

From the radiological point of view, the following investigations are undertaken:

- CT scan with 3D reconstruction
- MRI

*Natural history of sincipital encephalocele*

Small frontonasal or nasoethmoidal encephalocele may go undetected as they are compatible with normal life. If the covering of the sac is ulcerated then chances of infection doubles and this could be a bad prognostic factor.

*Other factors with unfavorable prognosis*

- Development of hydrocephalus
- Presence of other congenital cerebral anomalies

*Surgery*

The objective of surgery is to reduce the abnormal tissue, respect what the surgeons may consider as normal and to close the dura mater at the level of the bone dural with dural graft. It may seem extreme to reduce the tissue that appear on MRI as being normal; nonetheless, the histopathology confirms repeatedly that the tissue embedded within the sac is abnormal. In one of our patients there was presence of diffusely positive GFAP indicating glial cell lines, along with synaptophysin and neurofilament-positive neurons. In another patient the pathologist described presence of disorganized mass of neuroglial tissue with evidence of astrocytic gliosis along with presence of fibrous tissue.

## Atretic encephalocele

*Definition*

Atretic encephaloceles are a *forme fruste* of cephalocele. But this term should not lead us to conclude that it is a truly benign condition compared to other encephaloceles, as other associated anomalies of the CNS can be present and this is not uncommon in the presence of an atretic encephalocele.

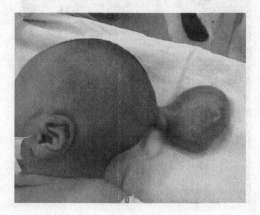

## Incidence

They represent about 38–50% of all encephaloceles. No known genetic defect or teratogenic defect has been implicated in the origin of atretic encephalocele. They are usually midline lesions, situated just underneath the scalp tissue and contain meninges, remnants of glial and neuronal tissue. At times they are mostly cystic lesions, representing pouching of meninges containing fluid with absence of any neural tissue. From the above illustration it is evident that the morphology of the lesion can be variable at times, being flat or nodular, or a purely cystic lesion. Among the differential diagnosis of an atretic encephalocele, dermoid cyst and sinus pericranii are the most common differentials to be considered.

## Clinical manifestations

In clinical encounter with a case of atretic encephalocele, the treating physician should look for presence of other associated anomalies. These anomalies include agenesis of the corpus callosum, holoprosencephaly, gray matter heterotopia, and Dandy–Walker malformation. The cerebro-oculo-muscular syndrome, Walker–Warburg, has also been described in children with atretic encephalocele. The MRI shows that the sac contains mostly fluid and suggests a remnant of embryonic neural tissue. This characteristic has led physicians to ignore other conditions listed above.

244                           *Neural Tube Defects*

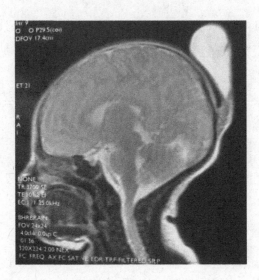

## Pathogenesis

The mechanism of origin of this atretic encephalocele is similar to the pathogenesis of encephaloceles in other locations, which is described briefly here. The mesoderm fails to interpose between the neuroectoderm and the cutaneous ectoderm. If the defect is small then the result is a meningocele, as illustrated in the patient above. It is presumed that there is intrauterine regression of the encephalocele, subsequently resulting in an atretic encephalocele.

## Treatment

Surgery is indicated to allow closure of the skull by reducing the wedge between the parietal bones. When the lesion is along the sagittal plane the relation of the lesion with the sagittal sinus needs to be determined.

## Occipital encephalocele

This encephalocele has the most menacing appearance. But by appearance alone we should not be prepared to cast judgment on the outcome of the child. Three cases of identical diagnosis but with very different characteristics are presented below.

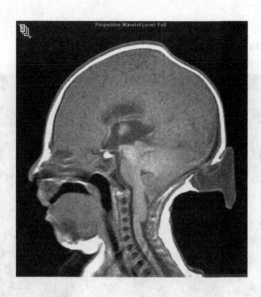

(1) The presence of a defect in the occipital bone is seen. It represents an occipital encephalocele. Partial agenesis of corpus callosum and colpocephaly is noted. The radiologist notes the presence of low lying cerebellar tonsils with descent of the tonsils being 5 mm below the foramen magnum. There is molding of the medulla with the tonsillar tissue and a prominent cervical medullary kink is also present. Small posterior fossa, tectal beaking with enlarged massa intermedia are the rest of the findings observed.

(2) Two-year-old female child with gross developmental delay and prenatally diagnosed occipital encephalocele.

*MRI*

- Presence of 2.2 cm defect in the occipital skull.
- Presence of 8.7 × 8 × 11 cm of occipital encephalocele containing brain content, CSF and cyst which has a distinct fluid level indicating blood products.
- Herniation of posterior fossa elements, mainly cerebellum, into the sac.
- Left cerebral hemisphere is smaller, probably also herniated into the sac.

- Distortion of brain stem structure.
- Right lateral ventricle is distended.

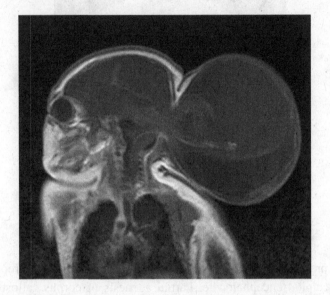

(3) Nine-month-old child. Presented with large encephalocele, with cere-
    bral content in the sac, the child nonetheless had a normal development
    after surgery. Before the surgery it was difficult for her to control the
    position of her head.

*Definition*

Occipital encephalocele is a type of encephalocele, where there is herniation
of the intracranial contents through a congenital bony defect located
above the external occipital protuberance, i.e. between the lambda and the
foramen magnum. When the bony defect involves not only the foramen
magnum but extends to the first cervical laminae, the lesion is then
called *occipitocervical encephalocele*. When occipital or occipitocervical
encephalocele is associated with hindbrain herniation along with other
findings of Chiari malformation, it is known as *Chiari type III*.

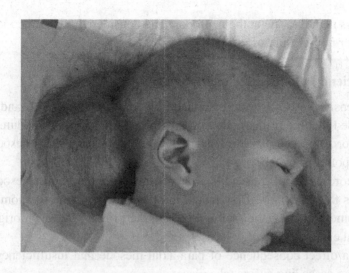

- Most occipital encephaloceles are sporadic in nature but incidences of familial occipital encephalocele have been reported with autosomal dominant pattern of inheritance.
- 4–7% of children have multiple neural tube defects, which means that there is encephalocele concurrent with presence of spinal dysraphism like myelomeningocele.
- 50% of afflicted children have other systemic abnormalities present.
- Chromosomal abnormalities, especially aneuploidy, have been reported in the literature with an incidence of 5–17%.

*Embryology*

From the embryological point of view, occipital encephalocele represents an anomalous development of the skull base involving the basichondrocranium and the membranous neurocranium.

*Embryological theories of encephalocele*

**Non-closure of anterior neuropore**
Patten *et al.* considered the non-closure of the anterior neuropore as the main pathogenesis of encephalocele. In his study, Pattern reported the presence

of excess neural tissue at the neuropore and considered this as the inciting factor for non-closure of neural tube.

## Insufficiency of para-axial mesoderm

An extensive research was undertaken by Marin-Padilla *et al.* and they concluded that the primary abnormality underlying cranium bifidum is in the abnormal development of axial skeleton from para-axial mesoderm. This hypothesis is elaborated here.

According to Marin-Padilla, early damage to the chordamesoderm, which is the precursor of para-axial mesoderm, could lead to anomalous development of the para-axial mesoderm, the primary defect in origin of occipital encephalocele.

As a direct consequence of para-axial mesodermal insufficiency, the following cascading events take place:

- Impaired longitudinal growth of axial skeleton
- Secondary impairment in formation and elevation of neural folds leading to dysraphism, which means failure of closure of the neural tube
- Overfolding or crowding of the normally developing notochord which underlies the shortened region of axial skeleton

*Possible teratogens in etiology of occipital encephalocele*

- Folic acid antagonist such as antiepileptic drugs
- Trypan blue (a chemical classified as a human teratogen)
- Vitamin A exposure in the first trimester
- Radiation exposure
- Possibility of rubella infection *in utero*
- Maternal gestational diabetes mellitus
- Maternal hyperthermia

*Pathology*

## Bony defects

Abnormal growth of the basichondrium may be due to restriction of its longitudinal growth more than its transverse growth, which results in a small posterior fossa. Evidence of abnormal development of basichondocranium is revealed by the following:

- Short basiocciput
- Narrow and funnel-shaped posterior fossa
- Presence of slight lordotic shape of occiput with respect to the axial skeleton
- Sharp downward bending of the petrous temporal bone
- Clivus at right angle to orbital wings of sphenoid
- Occasional agenesis of arch of atlas
- Presence of cleft palate

## Gross pathology of intracranial contents

Common pathological findings in occipital encephalocele include morphological abnormality associated with displacement of the mesencephalic structures and the roof of diencephalons. This point of displacement of the cerebral structures corresponds to the location of the anterior neuropore.

Thus it can be concluded that the defect in the origin of occipital encephalocele comes from failure of closure of the anterior neuropore. A striking similarity with Chiari malformation is evident and these common features lead many embryologists to rethink the pathophysiology of the origin of Chiari malformation.

**Cerebral hemispheres**: Herniation of cerebral contents is always asymmetrical with the cortex of the herniated part showing extensive vascular lesion in the form of old and recent infarction. However, the cerebrum has normal cytoarchitecture with only the hippocampus allocortex showing some abnormalities.

**Ventricular system**: The ventricles remain compressed or distorted with a tendency to fuse whenever the walls come into apposition.

**Basal ganglia**: Few abnormalities are seen in the basal ganglia with occasional presence of fused thalami.

**Optic pathways** are stretched with presence of atrophic optic chiasm and tracts.

**Commissural system**: Agenesis of anterior commissure, septum pellu-cidum and fornical system are seen.

**Hypothalamic area**: Considerable distortion of preoptic area was noted.

**Brain stem**: Hindbrain is severely affected and distorted with an abnormal plexus of vessels surrounding mainly the cervical cord and the lower medulla. Presence of diffuse areas of fibrillary gliosis is seen. Markedly distorted motor tracts with relative preservation of sensory pathways are also observed. Cerebellar peduncles are replaced by gliotic tissue.

**Cerebellum**: Cerebellum is mostly rudimentary with absence of vermis in all cases.

**Spinal cord**: Spinal cord is distorted with side-to-side compression conforming along the lines of stress. However, there is relative sparing of the posterior horns of the cord with absence of recognizable pyramidal tracts. All cords have hydromyelia.

### Clinical manifestation

Occipital encephalocele is usually detected right after birth due to the presence of a mass lesion attached to the skull base or at times extending to the nape of the neck. The neonatologist is usually called for evaluation of such a mass, which is described here.

### Inspection

- Midline mass
- Located above the external occipital protuberance
- Covered by atrophic or alopecic skin; occasionally there is an angioma present in the overlying skin
- Base of mass covered with hair

### Palpation

- Pulsations can be felt
- Cough impulse present
- Fluctuant mass

*Diagnostic imaging*

## Antenatal diagnosis of occipital encephalocele

By the second trimester, a sac-like protrusion is seen on the fetal ultrasound with a thin curvilinear echogenic structure representing the meningeal outer margin of the encephalocele. Target sign is seen with the tongue-like protrusion into the sac which indicates the brain tissue herniating into the encephalocele.

**MRI**: shows not only the defect, but also the contents of the sac and other associated anomalies.

**MRA**: shows the relation of blood vessels to the encephalocele defect.

**CT scan**: Bony defects are better seen.

*Differential diagnosis*

Causes of occipital swelling in a newborn:

- Cephalohematoma
- Caput succedaneum (crosses suture line)
- Subgaleal hematoma (crosses suture line)
- Traumatic hematoma with underlying skull fracture
- Hemangioma (usually not manifested at birth)
- Rare cases like dermoid cyst/congenital neoplasm such as teratoma

*Clinical outcome of patients with occipital encephalocele*

Long-term prognosis depends on:

- Amount of neural tissue in the sac
- Presence of microcephaly

A giant encephalocele is when the encephalocele is larger than the head size. When the amount of brain in the sac exceeds that in the cranium, the prognosis is bad. About 60–70% of posterior encephalocele will require insertion of ventriculoperitoneal shunt for hydrocephalus. Intelligence depends on the degree of neural tissue in the sac while neurological outcome depends on the development of hydrocephalus.

## Treatment

As in any other encephalocele, the objectives are similar. Reduce the sac to the level of the skull, remove the abnormally developed cerebral tissue, close dura mater and if needed place a ventriculoperitoneal shunt for hydrocephalus.

Often the skull defect is not very big, even when the diameter of the sac is very large. In many cases it is enough for the bone to heal and to have its edges freed from dura and periosteal adhesions. In some other cases it is necessary to reconstruct the defect ideally with autologous bone.

## Syndromes associated with occipital encephalocele

Occasionally occipital encephalocele may be part of a genetic syndrome as described here:

| Name of syndrome | Frequency | Striking clinical features | Inheritance |
| --- | --- | --- | --- |
| Meckel syndrome | 80% | Polydactyly, polycystic kidney, ocular defects cardiac anomalies, orofacial clefting and ambiguous genitalia. | Autosomal recessive |
| Pseudo-Meckel syndrome | Not known | Arnold-Chiari, corpus callosum absent, cardiac anomalies, cleft palate, club foot, hammer toes. | Translocation (3p) |
| Knobloch syndrome | Not known | Vitreoretinal degeneration, high myopia, retinal detachment but normal intelligence. | Autosomal recessive |
| Von Voss syndrome | Not known | Aplasia of corpus callosum, hypoplastic olives and pyramids, phocomelia, urogenital anomalies, thrombocytopenia. | Autosomal recessive |
| Warfarin syndrome | Uncommon | Nasal hypoplasia, optic atrophy, mental retardation, seizures, limb shortening, bone stippling, hydrocephalus. | Warfarin during pregnancy |

*(Continued)*

(*Continued*)

| Name of syndrome | Frequency | Striking clinical features | Inheritance |
|---|---|---|---|
| Chemke syndrome | Not known | Agyria, cerebellar dysgenesis, absent of cortical laminar structure, retinal dysplasia, corneal opacities, cataract. | Autosomal recessive |
| Cryptophthalmos syndrome | 10% | Extension of forehead skin to cover one/or both eyes, abnormal hairline, ear anomalies, syndactyly of hands or feet and genital anomalies. | Autosomal recessive |

Occipital encephalocele is associated commonly with urogenital anomalies, perhaps due to this embryological pathway which is described here in brief.

Primary abnormality in origin of occipital encephalocele lies in para-axial mesoderm.

- From intermediate mesoderm forms pronephros.
- Pronephros influences the mesonephros.
- Mesonephros in turn influences the Mullerian ducts formation (female genital organs at the level of third thoracic somite).
- Thus this explains the association of Mullerian ducts anomalies with encephalocele.

*Tumors associated with occipital encephalocele*

- Teratoma
- Lipoma

*Association of Mondini defect of cochlea and occipital encephalocele*

- Mondini defect is an important cause of congenital deafness, where cochlea has one and half turn.
- With the simultaneous development of the cochlea commencing on the fourth week of intrauterine life, the rostral limit of the neural tube closes.

- Ossification of the overlying ectoderm occurs, forming the bones of the skull.
- Mondini defect occurs when embryogenesis is arrested during the fourth to seventh week of intrauterine life.

*Other non-random association*

- The probability of Dandy–Walker syndrome is 11–16%. Dandy–Walker syndrome may represent compensation by the cyst for the raised intracranial pressure during fetal life.
- Diastematomyelia in 3% of patients.
- Kippell–Feil deformity.
- Corpus callosum defect such as lipoma or agenesis.
- Abnormal venous drainage of the great vein of Galen.
- Cardiac defects.
- Marfan syndrome and Ehlers–Danlos syndrome are acquired causes of occipital encephalocele due to abnormal connective tissue.

## Chiari type III

This is a rare malformation with very few cases reported in the literature which seems to be searching for a definition that goes beyond what it is not. In essence, the contents of the posterior fossa herniate through a low occipital or upper cervical bone defect.

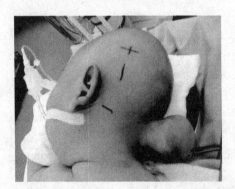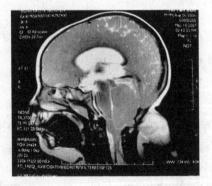

Although a myriad of CNS structures such as cerebellum, brain stem, and upper spinal cord can in theory be found in the sac, the cases described have two distinct presentations: basically normal examination or tetraparesis and apnea. The clinical picture can be inferred by analyzing the MRI. Hydrocephalus has been described in the great majority of the cases.

The predictors of outcome are similar to the one used for patients with encephalocele, which depends on the volume of neural tissue contained within the sac. Lesions of less than 5 centimeters in diameter do have a good outcome.

The timing of the surgery is determined by the general condition of the child. It is advisable to shunt the child if hydrocephalus is present, then wait for at least a year before attempting the repair of the sac. This conservative approach is recommended only if the skin that covers the sac is intact and there is no risk of meningitis.

Surgery is indicated for ablating the sac together with its contents. The dura mater needs to be repaired. Pre-operative or post-operative hydrocephalus needs to be shunted. The surgery should not worsen the pre-operative status of the patient, but it could happen that either the shift of the brain stem and upper cervical cord, or vascular insufficiency induced by the surgery, could lead to apnea and death.

## Suggested Readings

Bannister CM, Russell SA, Rimmer S, Thorne JA, Hellings S. Can prognostic indicators be identified in a fetus with an encephalocele? *Eur J Pediat Surg* 2000; **10**:20–23.

Barkovich AJ. Pediatric Neuroimaging. Raven Press, New York, 1990, pp. 108–113.

Cakirer S. Chiari III malformation: Varieties of MRI appearances in two patients. *Clin Imaging* 2003; **27**:1–4.

Caldarelli M, Rea G, Cincu R, Di Rocco C: Chiari type III malformation. *Child's Nerv Syst* 2002; **18**:207–210.

Cama A, Tortori-Donati P, Piatelli GL, Fondelli MP, Andreussi L: Chiari complex in children — neurological diagnosis, neurosurgical treatment and proposal of a new classification (312 cases). *Eur J Pediatr Surg* 1995; **5**:35–38.

Castillo M, Quencer RM, Dominguez R. Chiari III malformation: Imaging features. *AJNR* 1992; **13**:107–113.

Feuchtbaum LB, Currier RJ, Riggle S, Roberson M, Lorey FW, Cunningham GC. Neural tube defect prevalence in California (1990–1994): Eliciting patterns by type of defect and maternal race/ethnicity. *Genetic Testing* 1999; **3**:265–272.

Hedlund G. Congenital frontonasal masses: Developmental anatomy, malformations, and MR imaging. *Pediatr Radiol* 2006; **36**(7):647–662.

Holm C, Thu M, Hans A, Martina M, Silvia GS, Moritz S, Wolfgang M. Extracranial correction of frontoethmoidal meningoencephaloceles: Feasibility and outcome in 52 consecutive cases. *Plast Reconstr Surg* 2008; **121**(6):386e–395e.

Hoving EW. Nasal encephaloceles. *Child's Nerv Syst* 2000; **16**:702–706.

Lo BW, Kulkarni AV, Rutka JT, Jea A, Drake JM, Lamberti-Pasculli M, Dirks PB, Thabane L. Clinical predictors of developmental outcome in patients with cephaloceles. *J Neurosurg Pediatr* 2008; **2**:254–257.

Martinez-Lage JF, Poza M, Sola J, Soler CL, Montalvo CG, Domingo R, *et al.* The child with a cephalocele: Etiology, neuroimaging, and outcome.

Mayr U, Aichner F, Menardi G, Hager J. Computer-tomographical appearances of Chiari malformations of the posterior fossa. *Z Kinderchir* 1986; **41**:33–35.

Menezes AH. Neurological surgery, syringomyelia, Chiari malformations, and hydromyelia. 3rd ed, Vol 2. Youmans JR (Ed), Saunders, Philadelphia, 1990; pp. 1421–1459.

Meanley J Jr, Dzenitis AJ, Hockey AA. The prognosis of encephaloceles. *J Neurosurg* 1970; **32**:209–218.

McLone DG. Congenital malformations of the central nervous system. *Clin Neurosurg* 2000; **47**:346–377.

McLaurin RL. Parietal encephaloceles. *Neurology* 1964; **14**:764–772.

Muzumdar M, Gandhi R, Fatterpurkar S, Goel A. Type III Chiari malformation presenting as intermittent respiratory stridor: A neurological image. *Pediatr Nerosurg* 2007; **43**: 446–448.

Oakes WJ. Chiari malformations and syringomyelia. Wilkins RH, Rengachary SS: Principles of Neurosurgery, ed 2. London, Wolfe, 1994, Chap 9, pp 1–18.

Peter JC, Fieggen G. Congenital malformations of the brain — a neurosurgical perspective at the close of the twentieth century. *Child Nerv Syst* 1999; **15**:635–645.

Suwanwela C, Suwanwela N. A morphological classification of sincipital encephaloceles. *J Neurosurg* 1972; **36**:201–211.

Shokunbi T, Adeloye A, Olumide A. Occipital encephaloceles in 57 Nigerian children: A retrospective analysis. *Child's Nerv Syst* 1990; **6**:99–102.

# Chapter 23

# Hydrocephalus

Hydrocephalus is a pathology with no clear boundaries. It could be secondary to a brain tumor or meningitis, congenital in nature, complicating some patients with Chiari type I but not all of them, and patients can also be found with some NTDs.

Hydrocephalus is a condition that is perceived by patients, families and physicians as a setback, when in reality if treated proactively, after accepting that it is present, the patient can benefit from opportune derivation of the CSF.

The traditional definition states that hydrocephalus is the progressive enlargement of the lateral ventricles. A great majority of cases are secondary to some obstruction to the flow of CSF from the site of production, mostly from the lateral ventricles, to the site of absorption, the Pacchioni's granulations. In patients with MMCL, the CSF flow is blocked either at the level of the aqueduct by a congenital narrowing of the passage between the III and IV ventricles, or at the exit from the IV ventricles by the descended cerebellar tonsils that constitute an important part of the Chiari II complex.

But in patients with encephaloceles the source of the obstruction varies. In few cases there is associated descend of the cerebellar tonsils, in others the subarachnoid space is compromised due to traction and dislodgement provoked by the displacement of part of the brain outside the skull.

The pathophysiology of hydrocephalus as presented in conventional pediatric textbooks conveys the impression that the noxious effects of intracranial pressure are rapidly progressive and that if not treated on time the patient will die. This is true, but what is also true is that hydrocephalus exerts its effects in a more insidious manner. The shunt may not be fully obstructed, allowing some CSF to flow out from the ventricles into the peritoneum. While this does not kill the patient, it continues to damage the brain. It does so by a two-fold mechanism, one that impairs the cerebral perfusion pressure. We understand that:

$$\text{Cerebral perfusion pressure} = \text{mean arterial pressure}$$
$$- \text{intracranial pressure}$$

In this fashion the cerebral tissue will be starved of oxygen and nutrients, thus its development will be impaired.

The partially increased brain volume also stretches the dura mater, stimulating its pain receptors and the patient has a lingering headache that is not impossible to bear but is annoying enough to impair the patient's daily performance.

These diffuse symptoms that do not fit into the classical idea of progression, deterioration and death sometimes confuse the attending physician. To further confuse the issue, the child has a head CT scan which shows that the ventricles have not changed in size and the wrong diagnosis of functioning shunt is stamped.

While a progressive enlargement of the lateral ventricle is unequivocal evidence of shunt failure, the stability of the ventricular size is not proof of a working shunt. The symptoms are the determining factors of a diagnosis in hydrocephalus and in any other branch of medicine. A wise motto coined by Dr H. Humphrey states: "whatever the CT scan shows, whatever mom says." Thus, any impairment in the child's performance in school, any decrease in motor function, and certainly restlessness or irritability should alert the treating physician of a less than perfectly functioning shunt. A child with NTD is already physiologically and anatomically handicapped. It is our responsibility to assure that every system works at its best.

Now, what is mentioned above is of accepted practice. There are neurosurgeons who stand correctly in my opinion, although I still personally do not do it, regularly revise their patients' shunt every so many years. Nonetheless, even after accepting that the subtleties of the shunt have to be watched, we are reluctant to place a shunt in a patient who has enlarged lateral ventricles.

The following image belongs to a child who has large lateral ventricles. This specific condition is called *colpochephaly*, defined as enlargement of the occipital horns. This is attributed to thinning of the occipital cortex or thickening of the frontal cortex, a characteristic observed in children with NTD.

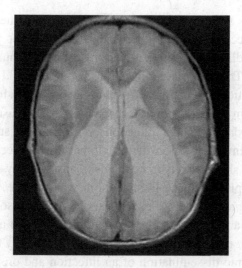

This particular child did not have the classical symptoms of hydrocephalus; no increase in head circumference, no drowsiness preceded by nausea and vomiting. But his cognitive development was not perfect. He had an occipital encephalocele, one of the small ones, the type that we assume will not dramatically impact the child's performance. So the question that follows is: Should we shunt this patient?

In favor of shunting we could emphasize that

$$\text{Tension} = \text{Pressure} \times 2\text{Area}$$

So if the ventricular area increased, then we have to infer that the tension exerted by the ventricles onto surrounding brain areas also increased. There is no study that confirms or refutes this assumption. Intuitively I will opt for shunting to reduce the tension. Here we have to acknowledge the intense, but not always justified, aversion that pediatricians and parents have against shunting.

The preferred place for diverting the CSF is the peritoneum. Usually the distal catheter placed in the peritoneal space has an extension of 30 centimeters, which is more than enough to compensate for the child's growth. The main difference in height between the child and his father is the extension of the legs, not the torso, thus rarely a prolongation of the peritoneal catheter has to be contemplated.

The atrium is also an alternative, but in this case as the distal catheter has to be at a precise position, otherwise it will be in the jugular vein or deep into the cardiac cavity, there is a strong chance of shunt failure when the child grows. Thus ventricular-atrial (VA) shunts should not be the first option for any patient. Sometimes VA shunts are an option for patients who have a peritoneum that does not absorb CSF adequately, usually seen after peritonitis secondary to shunt infection or Mitrofanoff surgeries. Shunt nephritis, the immune reaction of the glomeruli, has been described in patients with VA shunts for hydrocephalus of any etiology.

Finally, the pleural space is also another alternative. However, it is not effective in patients below eight years of age. It also indicated that the peritoneum fails to absorb fluid. As in the case with a VA shunt, the catheter has to be placed only when the fluid is absolutely normal. This is to prevent systemic dissemination of an infection and prevent the pleura from suffering the same phenomenon that occurred in the peritoneum.

In essence there are two types of shunt system: with antisiphon device and without it. The former has innovated along the years and today we even have the option of placing programmable valves. The latter is not widely used, although it is the preferred shunt for children in my institution. It is inexpensive, simple to place, requires very short surgical time, thus reducing the risk of infection and no mechanical parts. Without expanding on the merits of one or the other, we have not observed the supposed complications of shunts without antisiphon device. Often this simple shunt system is more popular because of its cost in developing nations, but physicians from any of the countries with lean healthcare budget should not feel that they are doing a disfavor to their patients.

Most shunt failure occur within the first six to 12 months and a comparative analysis was performed comparing shunt failure seen in myelomeningocele children vs. non-spina bifida cases. A higher rate of shunt malfunctions were seen in children with spina bifida with significant rate of shunt infections.

The symptoms of shunt failure are in essence those of increased intracranial pressure (ICP). If the child has an open fontanelle, or defect of an encephalocele, we may see and feel the brain bulging before the plethora of symptoms manifest. The ICP symptoms will manifest more rapidly in children with a closed fontanelle:

1. Headaches and irritability, if the child is mentally retarded and cannot verbalize pain and localize it. As expressed above this is secondary to the stretching of the dura mater.
2. Projective vomiting, supposedly secondary to pressure of the cerebellar tonsils over the brain stem.
3. And everything else that does not explain the drop in performance of the child.

The diagnosis is achieved through a combination of clinical judgment, radiological images and head CT scan. But a set of plain skull and abdominal X-rays can also inform if the shunt is short or if it has disconnected at some of its junctions.

The symptoms of an infected shunt are:

1. Fever of unexplained origin. In children with MMCL, urinary infection is the first culprit of increased body temperature.
2. Irritability and meningismus.
3. Drowsiness.
4. Acute abdominal pain, due to seeding of infected CSF in the peritoneal space.

While we always have to be suspicious of shunt infection, we have to remember that shunts do not get infected, surgeons are the ones who infected shunts. The further apart the date of surgery from the break of fever the less likely it is that the patient has an infected shunt. As urological procedures, which will be discussed later, expose the peritoneal catheter to the environment, I consider these procedures also a potential source of involuntary iatrogenia. I do not have a clear cut date but in general if the shunt was placed a year before I advise against taping the shunt for drawing CSF from the ventricle.

The reasons for increased frequency in shunt infection is perhaps secondary to the child having had a previous surgery on the CNS. With regards to shunt malfunction I am inclined to believe that while part of the problem resides in an imperfect anatomy to start with, there is also perhaps an element of sloppiness on the performing surgeon. I still have my share of shunt obstructions but since I started to thoroughly analyze the radiological studies of each individual patient before placing the shunt, I have a much better, but not yet perfect outcome than times in the past when such meticulousness was not always prevalent.

With regards to the activities that the child with a shunt can engage there is a wide range of opinions. I am of the idea that the presence of the shunt should not impede full physical activity in anybody. I think that almost every sport, including soccer, basketball, baseball and cricket, is inclusive in the range of permissible activities, with the exception of boxing or American football. Rugby is a toss up. My rationale is that the force that needs to be exerted on the skull which will affect the actual valve is so strong that it would be damaging in anybody independently of the shunt. I always emphasize that the eyes are actually more exposed to injury while playing team sports than the shunt system. Certainly I acknowledge that a serious head injury can become more serious because of the presence of a shunt, but this is a comparatively small risk to the enormous emotional advantage of not being restrained by another condition. In my experience, children and adults with NTD have an innate wisdom about what they can and cannot do.

## Chapter 24

# Multiple NTD

## Definition

Simultaneous presence of myelomeningocele at two or more sites or the presence of an encephalocele with a myelomeningocele is addressed as multiple NTDs. This is a very rare phenomenon with only few cases mentioned in the literature to date. The child below has an occipital encephalocele and a lumbar meningocele.

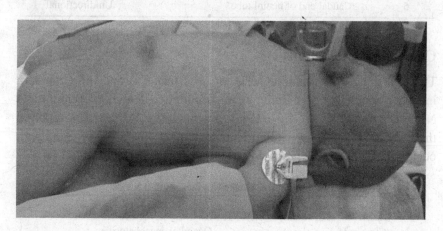

## Pathogenesis

According to the classical theory of neurulation, the primary closure of the neural tube commences from a single initiation site and then proceeds continuously in a bidirectional manner, i.e. towards the rostral and the caudal ends of the neural tube. This is called the "zipper-like closure of the neural tube". This hypothesis explains NTD as defective closure of anterior and posterior neuropores. However, it could not explain the whole gamut of NTDs, let alone the occurrence of multiple NTDs.

It was in 1993 that van Allen for the first time proposed the multisite closure of the neural tube. According to him, anencephaly, midline encephalocele and spina bifida are considered primary closure defects but lateral encephalocele is considered as a post-closure defect. The following are mention of various sites of closure and their associated pathologies. In the previous section where pathogenesis was discussed, the three-level theory was presented. Nonetheless, van Allen's five-site theory seems to fit this rare condition better.

| Closure site | Site of origin | Direction of progression |
|---|---|---|
| 1 | Mid-cervical level | Bidirectional |
| 2 | Junction between prosencephalon and mesencephalon | Bidirectional |
| 3 | Stomodeum | Unidirectional |
| 4 | Caudal end of rhombencephalon | Unidirectional |
| 5 | Caudal end of neural tube | Unidirectional |

## Clinical Manifestations

The occurrences of multiple NTD are less than 1% and most of them involve a double MMCL. Rarer are the occurrence of higher level multiple NTD as most cases are incompatible with life. However, it is reported that both VATER syndrome and Knobloch syndrome are associated with occipital encephalocele and MMCL.

| Sites of defective closure and associated NTDs | |
|---|---|
| **Site** | **Type of NTD** |
| Closure of 4 | Occipital encephalocele |
| Closures of 4 and 2 | Parieto-occipital encephalocele |
| Closures of 3 or 3 and 2 | Frontal encephalocele |
| Closures of 4 and 1 or Rostral 1 | Cervical MMCL |
| Caudal closure of 1 | Thoracolumbar MMCL |
| Closures of 1 and 5 | Lumbar MMCL |
| Closure of 5 | Lumbosacral MMCL or lipoma |

## Treatment

After birth, it has to be decided which lesion endangers the child and that is the one which has to be addressed first. In the case above the child was brought to the OR at four months of age and both defects were repaired simultaneously.

In another case reported the myelomeningocele was repaired at birth and the encephalocele/Chiari type II was repaired after shunting for hydrocephalus.

## Suggested Reading

Srinivas D, Sharma B, Mahapatra AK. Triple neural tube defect and the multisite closure theory for neural tube defects: Is there an additional site? *J Neurosurg Pediatr* 2008; Feb.; **1**(2):160–163.

## Chapter 25

# Genetic Syndromes Associated with Neural Tube Defects

## Introduction

Neural tube defects are the most common congenital disorders, second to only congenital cardiac defects. The etiology and genesis of neural tube defect are multifactorial and are associated with maternal and fetal risk factors. There is considerable evidence of environmental and genetic factors in the etiopathogenesis of NTD.

## Syndromes Associated with Cranial Defects

1. Omphalocele-Exstrophy-Imperforate anus-Spinal defects complex (OEIS)
2. Pentalogy of Cantrell
3. Amniotic band sequence
4. Limb-body wall complex
5. Meckel syndrome
6. Joubert syndrome
7. Skeletal dysplasia

| Name of syndrome | Type of NTD | Inheritance | Features of syndrome |
|---|---|---|---|
| 1. Omphalocele/ OEIS syndrome (omphalocele-exstrophy of bladder-imperforate anus-spinal defect) | Anencephaly/ myelomeningo-cele | Autosomal recessive — MTHFR-T mutation | • Ventral abdominal wall defect<br>• Absence of anterior bladder wall<br>• Anorectal anomaly<br>• Epispadias |

*(Continued)*

(*Continued*)

| Name of syndrome | Type of NTD | Inheritance | Features of syndrome |
|---|---|---|---|
| 2. Pentalogy of Cantrell | Posterior encephalocele/ anencephaly/ exencephaly myelomeningo-cele/ craniorachischi-sis | Trisomy-18 Rare syndrome | • Midline supraumbilical abdominal wall defect<br>• Midline sternal bone defect<br>• Defect in diaphragmatic pericardium<br>• Congenital cardiac defects |
| 3. Amniotic band syndrome | Encephalocele/ exencephaly/ anencephaly | Autosomal recessive/ teratogens like methadone | • Multiple craniofacial defects like cleft lip/cleft palate<br>• Autoamputation of digits<br>• Pseudosyndactyly<br>• Body wall defects |
| 4. Limb-body wall complex | Craniofacial defects — encephalocele | Sporadic | • Craniofacial defects<br>• Limb reduction anomalies<br>• Most are lethal |
| 5. Meckel–Gruber syndrome (dysencephalia splanchocystica) | Occipital encephalocele | Autosomal recessive (ciliary dysfunction) | • Bilateral renal cystic dysplasia<br>• Hepatic ductal proliferation<br>• Polydactyly<br>• Arnold Chiari<br>• Dandy–Walker syndrome |
| 6. Joubert Syndrome (cerebello-ocular renal syndrome) | Posterior encephalocele | Autosomal recessive (ciliary dysfunction) | • Hypoplasia of cerebellar vermis<br>• Retinal dystrophy<br>• Renal cyst and fibrosis<br>• Situs inversus (rare) |

(*Continued*)

| | Name of syndrome | Type of NTD | Inheritance | Features of syndrome |
|---|---|---|---|---|
| | *(Continued)* | | | |
| 7. | Skeletal dysplasia | Anencephaly/ posterior encephalocele | Sporadic | • Dwarfism<br>• Polycystic kidney |

## Syndromes Associated with Spinal Defects

1. Currarino syndrome
2. Sacral defect with anterior meningocele (SDAM)
3. Jarcho–Levin syndrome (spondylocostal dysostosis)
4. Lateral meningocele syndrome
5. VACTERL syndrome
6. Marfan syndrome
7. Neurofibromatosis type I

## Syndromes Associated with Spina Bifida

| | Name of syndrome | Type of NTD | Inheritance | Features of syndrome |
|---|---|---|---|---|
| 1. | Currarino syndrome | Anterior meningocele/ neurenteric cyst/ dermoid/ epidermoid cyst/ lipoma/teratoma | Sporadic | • Anorectal anomalies like imperforate anus/anal stenosis<br>• Horseshoe kidney/ duplex ureters<br>• Rectovaginal fistula<br>• Spinal cord tethering |
| 2. | Sacral defect with anterior meningocele (SDAM) | Anterior meningocele | Autosomal dominant | • Sacral agenesis<br>• Tethered spinal cord |
| 3. | Jarcho–Levin syndrome (spondylo-costal dysostosis) | Myelomeningocele/ lipomyelomeningo-cele/ diastematomyelia | Autosomal recessive | • Block vertebrae with kyphoscoliosis<br>• Rib anomalies<br>• Barrel-shaped thorax<br>• Opisthotonus head with short neck |

*(Continued)*

(*Continued*)

| Name of syndrome | Type of NTD | Inheritance | Features of syndrome |
|---|---|---|---|
| 4. Lehman syndrome (lateral meningocele syndrome) | Multiple thoracic and lateral meningocele | Autosomal dominant | • Craniofacial defects like hypertelorism, micrognathia<br>• Kyphoscoliosis<br>• Umbilical/inguinal hernia |
| 5. VACTERL syndrome | Vertebral anomalies | Sporadic | • V–vertebral defect<br>• A–anal atresia<br>• C–cardiac anomalies<br>• TE–Tracheo-esophageal fistula<br>• R–renal anomalies<br>• L–limb defects |
| 6. Marfan syndrome | Anterior or anterolateral thoracic meningocele | Autosomal dominant | • Cardiac defects like mitral valve prolapse, aortic aneurysm<br>• Ectopia lentis<br>• Skeletal defects |
| 7. Neurofibromatosis type I | Meningocele | Autosomal dominant | • Multiple neurofibroma<br>• CNS tumors vestibular schwannoma<br>• café au lait spots in skin |

# Less Common Syndromes Associated with NTD

1. Acrocallosal syndrome
2. X-linked NTD
3. Fetal valproate syndrome
4. DiGeorge syndrome
5. Waardenburg syndrome

# Glossary

---

**Aprosencephaly**: (Anencephaly/Iniencephaly/Encephalocele)

It is a severe form of cerebral malformation where both prosencephalic and diencephalic derivatives fail to develop. It presents with holoprosencephalic facies.

Treatment: None.

**Atelencephaly**: (Anencephaly/Iniencephaly/Encephalocele)

It is a lethal form of congenital cerebral malformation, where there is absence of any telencephalon-derived brain structures like the cerebrum and its related structures.

There is presence of a rudimentary prosencephalon. The cerebral hemispheres are either completely absent or reduced to a small discernible mass of tissue with absence of the ventricular system except for the fourth ventricle. However, the cerebellum and the posterior fossa contents are normal. There is always complete presence of the cranial vault.

The etiology of this congenital disorder is unknown. Sirenomelia is usually present in these patients without any presence of holoprosencephalic facies.

Treatment: None.

**Apert syndrome**: (Encephalocele)

Apert syndrome has two distinct features, which are bicoronal synostosis and maxillary hypoplasia, clinically seen as mid-facial hypoplasia.

The other craniofacial deformities seen in Apert syndrome are hypertelorism, exophthalmoses or proptosis and antimongoloid eyes or laterally down-sloping slant of eyes. Low-set ears accompanied by an abnormally small, flat nasal structure with a bulbous tip and syndactyly are common clinically detected features.

Progressive hydrocephalus is usually not a common feature of this syndrome. Intelligence in patients with Apert syndrome varies from normality to mental deficiency.

Clinical management is directed towards treatment of raised intracranial pressure, proptosis and eye care, craniofacial deformities and respiratory compromise. Upper and lower airway obstruction which can result in fatality in infancy should be taken care of appropriately.

The inheritance pattern of this syndrome is autosomal dominant with mutations in the gene encoding fibroblast growth factor receptor 2 (FGFR2), located on chromosome 10.

Treatment: Surgical repair.

- Craniofacial surgery with fronto-orbital advancement
- Hydrocephalus: Placement of ventriculoperitoneal shunt

**Corpus collosum agenesis**: (Myelomeningocele/Encephalocele)

It is a congenital condition which presents clinically with varied features ranging from neurocognitive deficits to minimally symptomatic cases. It is the associated conditions that determine the clinical picture. These include presence of hydrocephalus, cerebral palsy, genetic disorders and neural tube defects mainly in the form of encephalocele. Reported incidence is 1 to 4 per 1000 children with male predominance. The clues to early diagnosis in infancy are low-set ears, large head and poor muscle tone. The most common manifestation of agenesis of corpus callosum is seizures.

Treatment: Medicine for seizure.

**Craniosynostosis**: (Encephalocele)

It is defined as premature closure of one or more calvarial sutures, the junction between skull bones. Craniosynostosis is classified as *simple* when only one suture is fused, and *complex* or *compound* when two or more sutures are affected.

The consequence of this premature closure is development of an abnormal shape of head from restricted growth of bones perpendicular to the fused suture with increased growth for bones of open sutures.

Treatment: Release of the closed suture.

**Currarino syndrome**: (Myelomeningocele/Tethered cord/Syringomyelia)

This syndrome is characterized by the triad of sacral agenesis along with anorectal and urogenital anomalies and the presence of a presacral mass in the form of an anterior spinal dysraphism.

The syndrome has an autosomal dominant pattern of inheritance.

Other associated visceral malformations include duplicated ureters, duplicated kidneys, vesicoureteric reflux, a bicornuate uterus, rectovaginal fistula, aseptate vagina.

From the neurosurgical aspect of such cases, presence of anterior meningocele and neuroenteric cyst leading to spinal cord tethering should be of concern to the treating physician.

Treatment: Repair of the meningocele or untethering of cord.

**Dandy–Walker syndrome (DWM)**: (Iniencephaly/Encephalocele)

This is the most common congenital malformation affecting the cerebellum. DWM is characterized by cystic dilation of the IV ventricle associated with either complete or partial agenesis of the cerebellar vermis with an enlarged posterior fossa. The internal morphology is characterized by presence of an elevated tentorium along with the confluence of the straight and transverse sinuses.

The reported incidence of DWM is 1 case per 25,000 live births, accounting for 1–4% cases of hydrocephalus in children.

Clinical manifestation: Macrocephaly, hydrocephalus, hypertelorism, strabismus, psychomotor retardation.

Treatment: Management of DWM is directed towards treatment of hydrocephalus. Placement of ventriculoperitoneal shunt or fenestration of the posterior fossa cyst may be required.

**Holoprosencephaly**: (Iniencephaly)

This is a disorder of abnormal prosencephalic cleavage and results in incomplete development and abnormal septations of midline CNS structures. Most of the cases are sporadic in nature with few case reports of associated chromosomal anomalies present. Associated features include craniofacial clefts, hypotelorism and nasal malformations.

It may occur as an isolated abnormality or in association with other brain defects seen with multiple congenital syndromes.

**Hypertelorism**: (Encephalocele)

This occurs when the distance between the medial and the lateral orbital walls increased.

Treatment: Surgical (fronto-orbital correction).

**Hydrocephalus**: (Myelomeningocele/Syringomyelia/Encephalocele)

Hydrocephalus is a progressive disorder in which the cerebral ventricular system contains an excess amount of CSF and is dilated because of increased intracranial pressure. Hydrocephalus are classically divided in two types: *communicating hydrocephalus* (impaired absorption or excessive production) and *obstructive hydrocephalus*.

Treatment:

- Placement of ventriculoperitoneal shunt (VP shunt) for all types of hydrocephalus.
- Endoscopic third ventriculostomy (ETV) only in cases of obstructive hydrocephalus.

**Lissencephaly (agyria)**: (Iniencephaly/Encephalocele)

This is a disorder caused by molecular alterations of the genes that mediate the neuronal migration. Due to this impaired migration of neurons from the germinal matrix lining the ventricles, the six cortical layers do not form normally. The surface of the brain appears completely or partially smooth with loss or reduction of sulci. Lissencephaly may be caused by intrauterine infection and decreased placental perfusion failure. Although sporadic in origin, genetic autosomal recessive inheritance, or *de novo* translocations and deletions are also seen. Microcephaly develops in all patients with lissencephaly by the first year of life, although a minority of cases are microcephalic at birth.

Clinical manifestation: Hydrocephalus, epilepsy, psychomotor retardation, muscle tone alterations.

Treatment:

- Medical treatment for seizures.
- Hydrocephaly: Placement of ventriculoperitoneal shunt.

**Macrocephaly**: (Myelomeningocele/Encephalocele)

This is defined as an OFC greater than two standard deviations (SD) above the mean for a given age, sex, and gestation ($\geq$ 97th percentile).

Treatment: If hydrocephaly, ventriculoperitoneal shunt placement is required.

**Marfan syndrome**: (Encephalocele)

Marfan syndrome is a connective tissue disorder with an autosomal dominance pattern of inheritance. It presents with multisystem involvement which includes ocular, cardiovascular and musculoskeletal abnormalities.

Clinical symptoms: Common presentations include cardiac valvular disorders like aortic regurgitation or mitral valve prolapse and aortic dissection, dural ectasia, ocular abnormalities, and arachnodactyly.

Treatment: Cardiovascular management.

**Megalencephaly/Macrencephaly**: (Encephalocele)

It means enlargement of the brain parenchyma.

Treatment: None.

**Microcephaly**: (Anencephaly/Iniencephaly/Encephalocele)

This is referring to an occipitofrontal circumference of more than two standard deviations (SD) below the mean for a given age, sex and gestation (< 3rd percentile).

Treatment: None.

**Micrencephaly**: (Anencephaly/Iniencephaly/Encephalocele)

This means an abnormally small brain. Micrencephaly is a neuropathologic or radiological imaging diagnosis.

Treatment: None.

**Neuronal heterotopias**: (Iniencephaly/Encephalocele)

This constitutes neuronal migration. The heterotopias are defined as ectopic collections of normal neurons placed in an abnormal location and may involve any part of the cerebral hemisphere, i.e. between the ventricular wall and the cortex. Some may be located subcortically.

Clinical manifestation: Seizures.

Treatment: Antiepileptic drug therapy.

**Optic nerve**: (Anencephaly/Iniencephaly/Encephalocele)

*Optic nerve aplasia*

It is characterized by a complete lack of the optic nerve fibers, optic disc, retinal nerve fiber layer, ganglion cells, and retinal vasculature. It is an extremely rare anomaly with non-hereditary occurrence of unknown etiology.

Usually presents unilaterally. It is associated with other ocular malformations like cataract, retinal dysplasia, microphthalmia, anterior chamber angle malformation, anterior coloboma, and iris hypoplasia.

*Optic nerve hypoplasia*

It is the most common congenital optic disc anomaly characterized by presence of a hypoplastic disc which is small, pale and surrounded by a yellowish halo with ring of pigmentation at the border. This sign is described as a double-ring sign.

Major retinal blood vessels may appear tortuous with anomalous branching patterns. Visual function can vary from 20/20 to no light perception. However, it is a non-progressive disorder. Thus, visual prognosis in an infant can be variable.

*Optic disc coloboma*

The malformation refers to a notch, gap, hole, or fissure in any of the ocular structures. Coloboma is frequently associated with microphthalmia. Coloboma generally results from failure of the fetal or choroidal fissure to close during the fifth to seventh week of fetal life. This is the period between the invagination of the optic vesicle and the closure of the fetal fissure. Almost any ocular structure may be involved, including the cornea, iris, ciliary body, zonule (lens), choroid, retina, optic disk, and/or optic nerve. It is classified as typical when the inferonasal quadrant is involved and atypical when located anywhere other than the inferonasal quadrant.

This fissure or cleft appears as a sharply defined, white, inferiorly decentered excavation of the optic on fundus examination. Optic disc colobomas occur unilaterally or bilaterally with equal frequency and may be sporadic or inherited. The defect may extend inferiorly and involve the adjacent retina and choroid; rarely, the entire disc is affected. Visual loss is variable and difficult to predict based on disc appearance. Macular sparing by associated chorioretinal coloboma is the best predictor for good visual acuity. Colobomas of the iris and ciliary body often coexist with optic disc coloboma.

Treatment: Eye surgery.

### Optic disc drusen

They are described as multilobulated, globular concretions composed of mucoprotein matrix with acid mucopolysaccharides and ribonucleic acid that calcify progressively. In most cases visual acuity is well preserved; visual fields, however, are often abnormal and can further deteriorate without the patients being aware of these defects. On fundus examination, optic disc drusen appear as multiple round to irregular, whitish-yellow dots or granules within the nerve substance, on the surface of the disc, and occasionally in the peripapillary retina.

Treatment: No effective treatment has been established.

### Pachygyria (macrogyria): (Iniencephaly)

This is a developmental malformation characterized by a reduction in the number of sulci of the cerebrum and is often seen in association of lissencephaly.

Clinical manifestation: Microcephaly, epilepsy, and psychomotor retardation.

Treatment: Medical treatment for seizures.

### Polymicrogyria (microgyria, micropolygyria): (Iniencephaly)

This is the most common form of neuronal migrational disorder resulting in disruption of appropriate cortical organization. It is characterized by presence of microconvolutions separated by numerous or excess of small sulci. The pathology behind this malformation is the anomalous migration of neurons to the cerebral cortex and failure to acquire proper neuronal connections.

Clinical manifestation: Epilepsy, psychomotor retardation.

Treatment: Medical treatment for seizures.

### Schizencephaly: (Iniencephaly)

This is a congenital cerebral malformation where there is abnormal neuronal migration characterized by presence of clefts in the cerebral gray matter which may or may not communicate with the ventricles.

Clinical manifestation: Microcephaly, epilepsy, global psychomotor retardation, motor deficit.

Treatment: Antiepileptics.

**Scoliosis**: (Myelomeningocele/Lipomyelomeningocele/Diastematomyelia/ Caudal Regression Syndrome/Tethered Cord/Syringomyelia)

This is a structural alteration defined as a lateral curvature of the spine that is usually accompanied by some degree of rotation of the spine. By convention, a curvature greater than 10° (measured by Cobb angle) is defined as scoliosis.

Clinical presentation: Asymmetry of the shoulders, scapulae or hips. Patients with severe scoliosis may develop restrictive pulmonary disease.

Treatment: Cobb angles of <20° may be treated conservatively, 20–40° bracing, ≥ 50° surgery.

Treatment: Observation, bracing, or surgery.

**Tinnitus**: (Encephalocele)

Tinnitus is defined as a perception of sound in the absence of an external source of sound. The symptom can start in one or both ears. The sound is often perceived as buzzing, ringing, or hissing, although it can be a combination of all in the form of a disturbing noise. Tinnitus is more common in men than women and the prevalence of tinnitus increases with age.

**Vater syndrome**: (Caudal Regression Syndrome/Tethered Cord)

It is a constellation of defects presenting with congenital anomalies of the vertebral column/anal atresia/tracheoesophageal fistula/radial limb reduction and renal defect.

Treatment: Surgical correction of the malformations.

# Index

*Neural Tube Defects*

*Index*                                                                    283